Autism Spectrum Disorder Across the Lifespan: Part I

Editors

ROBERT WISNER-CARLSON
SCOTT R. PEKRUL
THOMAS FLIS
ROBERT SCHLOESSER

CHILD AND ADOLESCENT PSYCHIATRIC CLINICS OF NORTH AMERICA

www.childpsych.theclinics.com

Consulting Editor
TODD E. PETERS

April 2020 • Volume 29 • Number 2

ELSEVIER

1600 John F. Kennedy Boulevard ● Suite 1800 ● Philadelphia, Pennsylvania, 19103-2899

http://www.theclinics.com

CHILD AND ADOLESCENT PSYCHIATRIC CLINICS OF NORTH AMERICA Volume 29, Number 2
April 2020 ISSN 1056–4993, ISBN-13: 978-0-323-73309-0

Editor: Lauren Boyle
Developmental Editor: Kristen Helm

Child and Adolescent Psychiatric Clinics of North America (ISSN 1056-4993) is published quarterly by Elsevier Inc., 360 Park Avenue South, New York, NY 10010-1710. Months of issue are January, April, July, and October. Business and Editorial Offices: 1600 John F. Kennedy Boulevard, Suite 1800, Philadelphia, PA 19103-2899. Periodicals postage paid at New York, NY and additional mailing offices. Subscription prices are $338.00 per year (US individuals), $661.00 per year (US institutions), $100.00 per year (US & Canadian students), $388.00 per year (Canadian individuals), $804.00 per year (Canadian institutions), $446.00 per year (international individuals), $804.00 per year (international institutions), and $200.00 per year (international students). International air speed delivery is included in all *Clinics* subscription prices. All prices are subject to change without notice. **POSTMASTER:** Send address changes to *Child and Adolescent Psychiatric Clinics of North America*, Elsevier Health Sciences Division, Subscription Customer Service, 3251 Riverport Lane, Maryland Heights, MO 63043. **Customer Service: 1-800-654-2452 (U.S. and Canada); 314-447-8871 (outside U.S. and Canada). Fax: 314-447-8029.** E-mail: JournalsCustomer Service-usa@elsevier.com **(for print support) or** journalsonlinesupport-usa@elsevier.com **(for online support).**

Reprints. For copies of 100 or more of articles in this publication, please contact the Commercial Reprints Department, Elsevier Inc., 360 Park Avenue South, New York, New York 10010-1710 Tel.: 212-633-3874; Fax: 212-633-3820, E-mail: reprints@elsevier.com.

Child and Adolescent Psychiatric Clinics of North America is covered in *MEDLINE/PubMed (Index Medicus), ISI, SSCI, Research Alert, Social Search, Current Contents,* and *EMBASE/Excerpta Medica.*

Contributors

CONSULTING EDITOR

TODD E. PETERS, MD, FAPA
Medical Director, Child and Adolescent Services, Chief Medical Information Officer (CMIO), Sheppard Pratt Health System, Sheppard Pratt Physicians PA Clinical Operations Liaison, Baltimore, Maryland, USA

EDITORS

ROBERT WISNER-CARLSON, MD
Medical Director, Neuropsychiatry Outpatient Program, Director, Adult Developmental Neuropsychiatry Clinic, Senior Psychiatrist and Service Chief, Adult Inpatient Intellectual Disability and Autism Unit, Clinician Investigator, Sheppard Pratt Autism Registry, Chairman, Ethics Committee, Sheppard Pratt Hospital, Adjunct Assistant Professor, University of Maryland School of Medicine, Baltimore, Maryland, USA

SCOTT R. PEKRUL, MD
Service Chief, Child and Adolescent Inpatient Neuropsychiatric Unit, Sheppard Pratt Health System, Baltimore, Maryland, USA

THOMAS FLIS, MS, BCBA, LBA, LCPC
Senior Behavior Analyst, Behavioral Services Manager, Sheppard Pratt Health System, Baltimore, Maryland, USA

ROBERT SCHLOESSER, MD
Director, Point-of-Care Research and Innovation, Associate Chief Medical Information Officer, Sheppard Pratt Health System, Baltimore, Maryland, USA

AUTHORS

LAUREN AVELLONE, PhD
Research Associate, Department of Counseling and Special Education, Rehabilitation Research and Training Center, Autism Center for Excellence, School of Education, Virginia Commonwealth University, Richmond, Virginia, USA

ABIGAIL BANGERTER, DEdPsy
Clinical Research Manager, Janssen Research & Development, LLC, Titusville, New Jersey, USA

CLAIRE M. BROWN, BPsySc, GDipPsych
Deakin University, School of Psychology, Faculty of Health, Burwood, Victoria, Australia

NANETTE ELSTER, JD, MPH
Associate Professor, Neiswanger Institute for Bioethics, Loyola University Chicago Stritch School of Medicine, Maywood, Illinois, USA

AMY ESLER, PhD
Associate Professor, Department of Pediatrics, University of Minnesota, Minneapolis, Minnesota, USA

KATHLEEN A. FLANNERY, MEd
Regional Director of School Programs, Sheppard Pratt Health System, Towson, Maryland, USA

THOMAS FLIS, MS, BCBA, LBA, LCPC
Senior Behavior Analyst, Behavioral Services Manager, Sheppard Pratt Health System, Baltimore, Maryland, USA

ELIZABETH A. LAUGESON, PsyD
Associate Clinical Professor, University of California, Los Angeles, Los Angeles, California, USA

CHRISTINE T. MOODY, MA
University of California, Los Angeles, Los Angeles, California, USA

MICHAEL J. MORRIER, PhD, BCBA-D
Assistant Professor, Department of Psychiatry and Behavioral Sciences, Program Director, Child Behavioral Interventions, Emory Autism Center, Atlanta, Georgia, USA

SETH NESS, MD, PhD
Clinical Lead, Janssen Research & Development, LLC, Titusville, New Jersey, USA

GAHAN PANDINA, PhD
Senior Director, Janssen Research & Development, LLC, Titusville, New Jersey, USA

KAYHAN PARSI, JD, PhD
Professor, Neiswanger Institute for Bioethics, Loyola University Chicago Stritch School of Medicine, Maywood, Illinois, USA

MARKIAN PAZUNIAK, MD
Department of Child and Adolescent Psychiatry, University of Maryland Medical Center, Baltimore, Maryland, USA

SCOTT R. PEKRUL, MD
Service Chief, Child and Adolescent Inpatient Neuropsychiatric Unit, Sheppard Pratt Health System, Baltimore, Maryland, USA

CATHERINE E. RICE, PhD
Professor, Department of Psychiatry and Behavioral Sciences, Director, Emory Autism Center, Atlanta, Georgia, USA

ROBERT H. RING, PhD
Chief Executive Officer, Kaerus Bioscience Ltd, London, United Kingdom

CAROL SCHALL, PhD
Assistant Professor, Co-Investigator Project SEARCH Plus ASD Supports, Department of Counseling and Special Education, Rehabilitation Research and Training Center, Director of Technical Assistance, Autism Center for Excellence, School of Education, Virginia Commonwealth University, Richmond, Virginia, USA

CORY SHULMAN, PhD
Professor, Director of the Autism Center of the Hebrew University of Jerusalem, Paul Baerwald School of Social Work and Social Welfare, The Hebrew University in Jerusalem, Jerusalem, Israel

MARK A. STOKES, PhD
Associate Professor, Deakin University, School of Psychology, Faculty of Health, Burwood, Victoria, Australia

JOSHUA P. TAYLOR, MEd
Research Associate, Department of Counseling and Special Education, Rehabilitation Research and Training Center, Autism Center for Excellence, School of Education, Virginia Commonwealth University, Richmond, Virginia, USA

SARA URAM, LCSW-C
Clinical Social Worker, Adult Developmental Neuropsychiatry Clinic, Sheppard Pratt Health System, Baltimore, Maryland, USA

PAUL WEHMAN, PhD
Principal Investigator Project SEARCH Plus ASD Supports, Department of Counseling and Special Education, Director, Rehabilitation Research and Training Center, School of Education, Autism Center for Excellence, Virginia Commonwealth University, Professor, Department of Physical Medicine and Rehabilitation, School of Medicine, Richmond, Virginia, USA

ROBERT WISNER-CARLSON, MD
Medical Director, Neuropsychiatry Outpatient Program, Director, Adult Developmental Neuropsychiatry Clinic, Senior Psychiatrist and Service Chief, Adult Inpatient Intellectual Disability and Autism Unit, Clinician Investigator, Sheppard Pratt Autism Registry, Chairman, Ethics Committee, Sheppard Pratt Hospital, Adjunct Assistant Professor, University of Maryland School of Medicine, Baltimore, Maryland, USA

Contents

Erratum   xi

Preface: Autism Spectrum Disorder Grows Up   xiii

Robert Wisner-Carlson, Scott R. Pekrul, Thomas Flis, and Robert Schloesser

Diagnosis of Autism Spectrum Disorder Across the Lifespan   253

Cory Shulman, Amy Esler, Michael J. Morrier, and Catherine E. Rice

Although autism spectrum disorder (ASD) is one of the most common neurodevelopmental disorders it is also one of the most heterogeneous conditions, making identification and diagnosis complex. The importance of a stable and consistent diagnosis cannot be overstated. An accurate diagnosis is the basis for understanding the individual and establishing an individualized treatment plan. We present those elements that should be included in any assessment for ASD and describe the ways in which ASD typically manifests itself at various developmental stages. The implications and challenges for assessment at different ages and levels of functioning are discussed.

The Role of Diagnostic Instruments in Dual and Differential Diagnosis in Autism Spectrum Disorder Across the Lifespan   275

Cory Shulman, Catherine E. Rice, Michael J. Morrier, and Amy Esler

The heterogeneity inherent in autism spectrum disorder (ASD) makes the identification and diagnosis of ASD complex. We survey a large number of diagnostic tools, including screeners and tools designed for in-depth assessment. We also discuss the challenges presented by overlapping symptomatology between ASD and other disorders and the need to determine whether a diagnosis of ASD or another diagnosis best explains the individual's symptoms. We conclude with a call to action for the next steps necessary for meeting the diagnostic challenges presented here to improve the diagnostic process and to help understand each individual's particular ASD profile.

Current Approaches to the Pharmacologic Treatment of Core Symptoms Across the Lifespan of Autism Spectrum Disorder   301

Gahan Pandina, Robert H. Ring, Abigail Bangerter, and Seth Ness

There are no approved medications for autism spectrum disorder (ASD) core symptoms. However, given the significant clinical need, children and adults with ASD are prescribed medication off label for core or associated conditions, sometimes based on limited evidence for effectiveness. Recent developments in the understanding of biologic basis of ASD have led to novel targets with potential to impact core symptoms, and several clinical trials are underway. Heterogeneity in course of development, co-occurring conditions, and age-related treatment response variability hampers study outcomes. Novel measures and approaches to ASD clinical trial design will help in development of effective pharmacologic treatments.

Autism and Education   319

Kathleen A. Flannery and Robert Wisner-Carlson

> Determining the most effective strategies to educate children and youth
> with autism spectrum disorder (ASD) can be daunting. Dr Stephen Shore,
> an autism advocate who is on the spectrum, said, "If you've met one per-
> son with autism, you've met one person with autism." Individuals diag-
> nosed with ASD present with unique strengths and difficulties and
> experience characteristics of their disability in different ways. General
> and special educators must be prepared with a variety of evidence-
> based practices and instructional strategies to engage and educate stu-
> dents diagnosed with autism. This article discusses current methods,
> techniques, evidence, and controversies for educating individuals diag-
> nosed with autism.

The Transition to Adulthood for Young People with Autism Spectrum Disorder   345

Robert Wisner-Carlson, Sara Uram, and Thomas Flis

> The transition to adulthood for individuals with autism spectrum disorder is
> difficult and outcomes are suboptimal. Social cognition deficits and exec-
> utive dysfunction continue to be barriers to young people's success, lack
> of societal acceptance and loss of previous support can exacerbate the
> condition, and mental health issues increase. All areas of adult functioning
> are affected. To help manage the transition and improve outcomes for this
> population, psychiatrists and other health care providers need to be aware
> of the issues and possible interventions, including social skills training,
> educational transition programs, and supported employment programs.

Social Skills Training in Autism Spectrum Disorder Across the Lifespan   359

Christine T. Moody and Elizabeth A. Laugeson

> Social skills training programs for individuals with autism spectrum disor-
> der are effective in improving social competence, although effects are
> frequently not robust across all outcomes measured. When aggregating
> across the social skills training programs with the strongest evidence,
> common elements can be identified in both the treatment delivery method
> and the social skills content targeted. However, social skills training pro-
> grams continue to remain limited in their generalizability and scope. Exist-
> ing research has primarily tested programs designed for school-aged
> children with autism spectrum disorder, who have average or above
> average intellectual functioning.

**Competitive Integrated Employment for Youth and Adults with Autism: Findings
from a Scoping Review**   373

Carol Schall, Paul Wehman, Lauren Avellone, and Joshua P. Taylor

> A scoping review was conducted to map existing literature on effective in-
> terventions for competitive employment for individuals with autism spec-
> trum disorder. Empirical database searches were conducted. A filter for
> level of methodological rigor was implemented. A total of 25 articles met
> inclusion criteria. Findings were categorized by level of evidence. Findings
> revealed strong empirical support for a transition-to-work program called

Project SEARCH plus ASD Supports and traditional supported employment services. Receipt of specific vocational rehabilitation and transition services in high school were also identified as effective interventions. Recommendations per level of evidence are provided in more detail.

Transitioning from Adolescence to Adulthood with Autism Spectrum Disorder: An Overview of Planning and Legal Issues   399

Nanette Elster and Kayhan Parsi

The transition to adulthood is complex. It is defined by many objective and subjective milestones. Transition from adolescence to young adulthood is challenging for both neurotypical individuals and individuals with autism spectrum disorders. However, for autistic individuals, this transition is even more complicated and poses a range of legal and ethical considerations. This article discusses how existing legal and social constructs may exacerbate rather than diminish barriers and access for autistic adults and identifies current and potential legal and policy solutions to reducing current systemic barriers. This article ultimately supports a supported decision-making model for autistic adolescents transitioning into adulthood.

Intersection of Eating Disorders and the Female Profile of Autism   409

Claire M. Brown and Mark A. Stokes

There is a moderate degree of comorbidity between autism and eating disorders, particularly anorexia nervosa in female individuals. Research indicates that up to 30% of patients with anorexia are autistic, or display high levels of autistic traits. Frequently, an autism diagnosis is secondary to an eating disorder diagnosis, which brings concomitant issues into treatment efficacy and outcomes for both conditions. Less is known about comorbidity with other eating disorder subtypes. Autistic traits can impede standard approaches to eating disorder treatment. Treatment options and settings may need to be modified to better accommodate autistic female individuals.

Obsessive–Compulsive Disorder in Autism Spectrum Disorder Across the Lifespan   419

Markian Pazuniak and Scott R. Pekrul

Obsessive–compulsive disorder is a relatively common disorder seen in autism spectrum disorder across the lifespan. Many obsessive–compulsive disorder symptoms can present similarly to the core features of autism spectrum disorder and it is often difficult to differentiate between obsessive–compulsive disorder and stereotypic behaviors or restricted interests in autism spectrum disorder. However, there are differences between the 2 disorders. This article is a review of the current literature with the goal of helping the clinician to diagnose and treat obsessive–compulsive disorder in a patient with autism spectrum disorder.

CHILD AND ADOLESCENT PSYCHIATRIC CLINICS

FORTHCOMING ISSUES

July 2020
Autism Spectrum Disorder Across the Lifespan: Part II
Robert Wisner-Carlson, Scott R. Pekrul, Thomas Flis, and Robert Schloesser, *Editors*

October 2020
Measurement-Based Care in Child and Adolescent Psychiatry
Jessica Jeffrey, Eugene Grudnikoff, Barry Sarvet, and Rajeev Krishna, *Editors*

January 2021
Sleep Disorders in Children and Adolescents
Argelinda Baroni and Jessica Lunsford-Avery, *Editors*

RECENT ISSUES

January 2020
Psychosis in Children and Adolescents: A Guide for Clinicians
Ellen M. House and John W. Tyson, *Editors*

October 2019
Eating Disorders in Child and Adolescent Psychiatry
James Lock and Jennifer Derenne, *Editors*

July 2019
Depression in Special Populations
Warren Y.K. Ng and Karen Dineen Wagner, *Editors*

SERIES OF RELATED INTEREST

Psychiatric Clinics of North America
https://www.psych.theclinics.com/
Pediatric Clinics of North America
https://www.pediatric.theclinics.com/
Neurologic Clinics
https://www.neurologic.theclinics.com/

AACAP Members: Please go to www.jaacap.org for information on access to the Child and Adolescent Psychiatric Clinics. *Resident* Members of AACAP: Special access information is available at www.childpsych.theclinics.com.

THE CLINICS ARE AVAILABLE ONLINE!
Access your subscription at:
www.theclinics.com

Erratum

For the article on "The Prodrome of Psychotic Disorders: Identification, Prediction, and Preventive Treatment" in the January 2020 issue of *Child and Adolescent Psychiatric Clinics of North America* (Volume 29, Issue 1), an error occurred on page 61. In the first full paragraph, the first sentence should read, "At long-term follow-up, UHR patients have been reported to have mild-moderate psychosocial functioning on the group level (a social and occupational functioning assessment scale score of ~68)".

The online version of this issue has been corrected.

Child Adolesc Psychiatric Clin N Am 29 (2020) xi
https://doi.org/10.1016/j.chc.2019.12.006
1056-4993/20/© 2019 Elsevier Inc. All rights reserved.

Preface

Autism Spectrum Disorder Grows Up

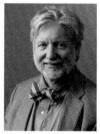 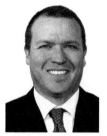 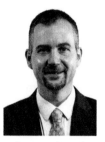 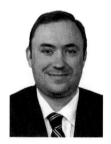

Robert Wisner-Carlson, MD   Scott R. Pekrul, MD   Thomas Flis, MS, BCBA, LBA, LCPC   Robert Schloesser, MD

Editors

Imagine arriving at early adulthood and yearning for independence, yet still struggling to comprehend what it means when someone raises their eyebrows or rolls their eyes, or even worse, being baffled when a coworker is offended by your bluntness. Most young adults with autism spectrum disorder (ASD) lack an understanding of basic social cues and the nuances of communication. They may find it difficult or impossible to behave in acceptable ways at a time of their life when societal expectations are rising and support services are declining.

Despite progress in the field of autism since its identification in 1943, given these intrinsic features of this lifelong disorder, it's not surprising that outcomes for individuals with ASD in postsecondary education, employment, and independent living remain woefully unacceptable in 2020. This special issue, published to coincide with World Autism Awareness Month in April, is dedicated to educating psychiatrists and other clinicians on how they can make a difference in the lives of a growing number of young people who present with this perplexing array of social and communication challenges. With prevalence close to 1.7% of the population, ASD is a complex neurodevelopmental disorder that all psychiatrists, pediatric and adult, need to learn more about.

Eighty-six years ago, Donald T. was born. His case, along with those of 10 other children, was reported in 1943 by Leo Kanner in *The Nervous Child* under the title "Autistic Disturbances of Affective Contact."[1] One year later, Hans Asperger published "Die 'Autistischen Psychopathen' im Kindesalter"[2] ("Autistic Psychopathy" in Childhood).[3] Once thought to be rare with a prevalence of 4.5 per 10,000,[4] ASD is now reported at a national rate of 1 in 59 children.[5] Individuals with ASD are at a higher risk of childhood and adult psychiatric problems[6] as well as medical comorbidities.[7,8] The outcomes for individuals with ASD are poor in terms of

Child Adolesc Psychiatric Clin N Am 29 (2020) xiii–xvi
https://doi.org/10.1016/j.chc.2020.02.001
1056-4993/20/© 2020 Published by Elsevier Inc.

childpsych.theclinics.com

reaching the milestones of adulthood.[9] This remains true when taking into account cognitive functioning levels. Individuals with ASD and Intellectual Disability (ID) function at lower levels compared with ID alone.[10] And individuals with high-functioning ASD have outcomes similar to Donald, who, in Kanner's 28-year follow-up report, was living at home with his parents, employed, but underemployed, with little ambition and only some social contacts.[11]

Today, ASD can be diagnosed as young as 2 years of age and is diagnosed throughout the lifespan, as reviewed by Shulman, Esler, Morrier, and Rice. Many diagnostic instruments are available in addressing the differential diagnosis of ASD and common dual diagnoses. There is no identified cure for ASD, though a strong research enterprise is pursuing this end. Many pharmacologic targets for the core symptoms of ASD are identified and are being actively researched, as reviewed by Bangerter, Pandina, Ring, and Ness. Children and youth with ASD require a special approach to education (see the article by Flannery and Wisner-Carlson in this issue). Early interventions for ASD have a significant impact on future outcomes. Because of this, more young adults with ASD are going to college and entering the workforce. They generally need additional assistance to do so, but such programs are increasingly supported by solid research. Social skills training, a mainstay of treatment reviewed by Moody and Laugeson, is effective in children and youth and is actively being developed for adults. Vocational research demonstrates that well-constructed supported employment programs are effective for individuals with ASD obtaining competitive integrated employment. This topic is reviewed by Schall, Wehman, Taylor, and Avellone.

The transition to adulthood, though, can be fraught with difficulties. ASD individuals require special approaches to overcome the social cognition and executive function problems that burden them, as reviewed by Wisner-Carlson, Uram, and Flis. Financial and legal planning for the transition is reviewed by Elster and Parsi, who explore ways to protect and support adult children in this transition, including shared decision making.

Brown and Stokes review the overlap of eating disorders and the female profile of autism. Pazuniak and Pekrul review obsessive compulsive disorder in ASD. These articles reflect the previously unexpected places ASD is encountered and the comorbid conditions of individuals with ASD. The higher risk of comorbid psychiatric and medical conditions drives further complexity and burden for individuals with ASD. Thus, the second issue of this 2-issue series on ASD Across the Lifespan will address these and other important issues.

At Sheppard Pratt Health System in Maryland, we are seeking to respond to an unprecedented demand for services by the ASD population. Approximately 1600 individuals with autism were served in the last year through our inpatient and outpatient programs and special education schools. The transition to adulthood is unquestionably the most challenging for these families. Because individuals with ASD do not necessarily present to specialists, it is incumbent on all providers to achieve a level of proficiency in evidence-based practices that will improve outcomes and the quality of life for these young adults. At the same time, we as clinicians need to advocate for more and better services that can help our patients become employed, continue their education, and live more independently.

Robert Wisner-Carlson, MD
Sheppard Pratt Health System
6501 North Charles Street
Baltimore, MD 21204, USA

Scott R. Pekrul, MD
Sheppard Pratt Health System
6501 North Charles Street
Baltimore, MD 21204, USA

Thomas Flis, MS, BCBA, LBA, LCPC
Sheppard Pratt Health System
6501 North Charles Street
Baltimore, MD 21204, USA

Robert Schloesser, MD
Sheppard Pratt Health System
6501 North Charles Street
Baltimore, MD 21204, USA

E-mail addresses:
RWisner-Carlson@sheppardpratt.org (R. Wisner-Carlson)
SPekrul@sheppardpratt.org (S.R. Pekrul)
tflis@sheppardpratt.org (T. Flis)
rschloesser@sheppardpratt.org (R. Schloesser)

REFERENCES

1. Kanner L. Autistic disturbances of affective contact. Nervous child. Nerv Child 1943;2(3):217–50.
2. Asperger H. Die "Autistischen Psychopathen" im Kindesalter. Arch Psychiatr Nervenkr 1944;117(1):76–136.
3. Asperger H. "Autistic psychopathy" in childhood. In: Frith U, editor. Autism and Asperger syndrome. Cambridge: Cambridge University Press; 1991. p. 37–92 [Frith U, Trans.].
4. Lotter V. Epidemiology of autistic conditions in young children. Soc Psychiatry 1966;1(3):124–35.
5. Baio J, Wiggins L, Christensen DL, et al. Prevalence of autism spectrum disorder among children aged 8 years—autism and developmental disabilities monitoring network, 11 sites, United States, 2014. MMWR Surveill Summ 2018;67(6): 1–23.
6. Lai M-C, Kassee C, Besney R, et al. Prevalence of co-occurring mental health diagnoses in the autism population: a systematic review and meta-analysis. Lancet Psychiatry 2019;6(10):819–29.
7. Levy SE, Giarelli E, Lee LC, et al. Autism spectrum disorder and co-occurring developmental, psychiatric, and medical conditions among children in multiple populations of the United States. J Dev Behav Pediatr 2010;31(4):267–75.
8. Davignon MN, Qian Y, Massolo M, Croen LA. Psychiatric and medical conditions in transition-aged individuals with ASD. Pediatrics 2018;141(Suppl 4):S335–45.

9. Howlin P, Magiati I. Autism spectrum disorder: outcomes in adulthood. Curr Opin Psychiatry 2017;30(2):69–76.
10. Bertollo JR, Yerys BE. More than IQ: executive function explains adaptive behavior above and beyond nonverbal IQ in youth with autism and lower IQ. Am J Intellect Dev Disabil 2019;124(3):191–205.
11. Kanner L. Follow-up study of eleven autistic children originally reported in. J Autism Child Schizophr 1971;1(2):119–45.

Diagnosis of Autism Spectrum Disorder Across the Lifespan

Cory Shulman, PhD[a],*, Amy Esler, PhD[b], Michael J. Morrier, PhD[c], Catherine E. Rice, PhD[c]

KEYWORDS

- Autism spectrum disorder • Diagnosis • Lifespan • Infancy and toddlerhood
- School age • Adult • Assessment

KEY POINTS

- Autism spectrum disorder (ASD) is one of the most common neurodevelopmental disorders.
- ASD is also one of the most heterogeneous conditions, making the identification and diagnosis of ASD a complex process.
- Symptoms of ASD vary over time, resulting diverse expressions of ASD at different developmental stages.
- The importance of a stable and consistent diagnosis cannot be overstated, given that an accurate diagnosis is the basis for understanding the individual and establishing an individualized treatment plan.

BACKGROUND

Over the last 30 years, the identification and definition of autism and related conditions have undergone a major transformation that has shaped the current autism spectrum.[1,2] The conceptualization of autism as a spectrum includes considering changes in autism across the lifespan, with the aging of the modern cohort of children and adolescents diagnosed on the autism spectrum moving into adulthood, and with younger children receiving an ASD diagnosis. As the definition of autism spectrum disorder (ASD) broadens, fundamental questions arise about the purpose, meaning, and function of an ASD diagnosis. Although many professionals note that the function of a diagnosis should be to inform intervention, the perspectives of self-advocates on the

[a] The Paul Baerwald School of Social Work and Social Welfare, The Hebrew University of Jerusalem, Mount Scopus, Jerusalem, 91905, Israel; [b] Division of Clinical Behavioral Neuroscience, Department of Pediatrics, University of Minnesota 2540 Riverside Ave S., RPB 550, Minneapolis, MN 55454, USA; [c] Emory Autism Center, 1551 Shoup Court, Department of Psychiatry & Behavioral Sciences, Emory University School of Medicine, Decatur, GA 30033, USA
* Corresponding author.
E-mail address: cory.shulman@mail.huji.ac.il

Child Adolesc Psychiatric Clin N Am 29 (2020) 253–273
https://doi.org/10.1016/j.chc.2020.01.001
1056-4993/20/© 2020 Elsevier Inc. All rights reserved.

childpsych.theclinics.com

Abbreviations	
ASD	Autism spectrum disorder
CDC	Centers for disease control and prevention
IDEA	Individuals with disabilities education act
PDD	Pervasive developmental disorders

spectrum have highlighted the disconnection between diagnosis and consideration of actual impact on the lives of those diagnosed.[3] Whether to inform intervention and supports, or to guide self-understanding and other-understanding of a person's way of experiencing the world, diagnosis is important in that it provides a guide for the person, their family, professionals, and the wider community within which the person is situated. The most important issue is whether the label helps inform the way the person engages with, learns from, and functions within the world they inhabit. Most articles on diagnosing ASD focus only on the mechanics of the process, including the signs indicating the need for an evaluation for autism and the tools and procedures for the diagnostic assessment. We will also position this discussion within a developmental framework, considering the implications of this assessment for the individual being assessed, as well as their family and other support systems in their life. Any diagnostic evaluation should seek to examine, understand, and facilitate meaningful engagement appropriate for that person's age, developmental level, and support context. In the case of autism, the fundamental question is whether people with an ASD diagnosis are able to attend to, engage with, learn from, and negotiate a world that is inherently socially mediated and therefore not completely understood by them, and to do this in a way that allows them to be safe and experience a positive quality of life. Thus, the diagnostic process cannot simply relate to the question "is this ASD or not?", but rather must gather data that can inform how to best identify the individual's strengths, facilitate supporting those strengths, and find the most appropriate methods to address the areas of need. This leads to working *with* people on the spectrum as partners, supporting their strengths, and understanding their experiences of the world.

"Autism" as a label describes a constellation of behaviorally identified criteria that cluster together in various patterns and severities. Its utility lies in describing and predicting behavior that does not fit the typical developmental progression. Kanner[4] and Asperger[5] first identified autism as a diagnostic classification over 75 years ago. Although Kanner's original description of autism was more widely known and influential in American psychiatry, it is possible that Kanner's and Asperger's work emerged almost simultaneously from their common Austrian professional milieu and through common colleagues.[6] Since Kanner's original description based on the profiles of 11 children with unusual social interaction, difficulties in communication, and focused and repetitive behaviors, much effort has gone into characterizing the diagnostic criteria of autism. The history of diagnosing autism reflects the need for specification of the phenomenological characteristics of autism, that is, the presence or absence of those behaviors that define it. This article presents the components of a diagnostic evaluation, indicating the elements that should be present at all ages and those which are age-specific, as well as possible additions and changes needed to address particular issues and enhance the diagnostic process. A Cory Shulman and colleagues' article, "The Role of Diagnostic Instruments in Dual and Differential Diagnosis in Autism Spectrum Disorder (ASD) Across the Lifespan," in this issue addresses the challenges encountered when adapting the diagnostic process and deciding which instruments to use that arise from the heterogeneity of autism due to the changing and broadening of diagnostic criteria, the diverse manifestations of ASD at different ages, and the need for differential dual diagnoses. This article takes a historical perspective when reviewing the diagnostic criteria, a developmental perspective in addressing the manifestations of ASD throughout the lifespan, and a multidisciplinary perspective in describing the diagnostic practice itself, presenting methods for fine-tuning the diagnostic process.

Although ASD is one of the most common neurodevelopmental disorders, with 1 in every 59 individuals in the United States identified as having ASD,[7,8] it is also one of the most heterogeneous conditions, making the identification and diagnosis of ASD a complex process. The multidimensional nature of the condition, as well as the variability of the symptoms and developmental changes that occur over the lifespan, contribute to the intricacy of the diagnostic evaluation. The importance of a stable and consistent diagnosis cannot be overstated, given that an accurate diagnosis is the basis for understanding the individual and establishing an individualized treatment plan. For example, it is widely accepted that early diagnosis is essential for tailoring early intervention strategies, which have been shown to result in better long-term outcomes for most children diagnosed with ASD.[9–12] In addition, access to service provision is often dependent on diagnosis.[13] Consequently, an age-appropriate and comprehensive diagnosis is the first step in understanding and treating ASD.

THE SEARCH FOR DIAGNOSTIC CLARITY: HISTORICAL PERSPECTIVE

When Kanner initially identified autism, it was characterized as a monolithic syndrome[14,15] that was a subtype of childhood schizophrenia, in which the core features were described as a profound lack of social understanding and a need for sameness. To attain singularity in autism, limit prevalence, and reduce heterogeneity, Kanner only diagnosed children without dysmorphic features and excluded those with very low IQ scores. Even with the constraints of Kanner's diagnostic criteria, it remained impossible to achieve consensus regarding the behavioral manifestations of "classical" autism, which was characterized by "autistic aloneness and a desire for sameness". Others followed Kanner in the attempt to define the behavioral characteristics necessary for an autism diagnosis. Rimland[16] believed that this diagnostic ambiguity could be addressed by gathering behavioral data concerning autism from parents and caregivers, and, thus, collected descriptions of autism using the E-2 questionnaire that he designed.[17] Instead of accumulating individual behavioral profiles, Wing and Gould[18] compiled a questionnaire and went into the field to investigate the specific characteristics of autism in institutions in the United Kingdom where such individuals with disabilities were living. As a result, Wing[19] posited that autism can be conceptualized as a "triad of impairments" (ie, a deficit in communication, a deficit in social interaction, and rigid thinking resulting in poor imagination). Additional explanations of ASD were based on possible causes. For example, Ornitz[20,21] suggested that autism is a disorder of sensory dysfunction, whereas Rutter[22] and Prior[23] initially believed that autism is fundamentally a cognitive deficit. Parents of children with autism also entered the dialogue concerning diagnostic criteria, reinforcing the need to describe the presence of abnormal behaviors characteristic of autism (eg, stereotyped movements) alongside the absence of typical behavior (eg, deficits in the social use of eye contact). The National Society for Autistic Children criteria for autism[24] appeared 3 years before the third edition of the *Diagnostic and Statistical Manual for Mental Disorders* (1980) in which the term pervasive developmental disorder (PDD) first appeared. In *DSM-III*, PDD was the umbrella term for 3 types of autism (early onset, childhood onset, and atypical), and represented an attempt to separate autism from schizophrenia, emphasizing the developmental base of autism.

The change in the conceptualization of ASD as a neurodevelopmental disorder, which appears in early childhood and continues throughout the lifespan, continued in subsequent editions of the Diagnostic and Statistical Manual of Mental Disorders (DSM; DSM-III-R, 1987; DSM-IV, 1994, DSM-IV TR, 2000; DSM-5, 2013). Currently, the diagnostic criteria for ASD are based on the fifth edition of the DSM,[25] and address some the challenges of diagnosing ASD that have arisen over the years. The changes in the newest edition are based on research findings and the decision that diagnoses should rely on information collected through the use of standardized diagnostic instruments, resulting in a reliable and valid diagnostic category.[26] The most outstanding change is expressed in the inclusion of all 5 of the distinct PDDs that appeared in the DSM-IV[27,28] in one overarching category of autism spectrum disorder. Thus autistic disorder, Asperger disorder, Rett disorder, childhood disintegrative disorder, and PDD not otherwise specified no longer exist as diagnostic subtypes, eliminating the need for differential diagnosis within the autism spectrum. In addition, the DSM-5 diagnostic criteria for ASD moved from a triad of impairments (impairments in social interactions, communication and behavior) to a dyad of impairments by combining the social and communication domains into a domain of impairments in social communication. Another significant change is the necessity of meeting all 3 of the social communication criteria, so that all individuals with a diagnosis of ASD have a core of similar impairments in social communication. Additional difficulties in social interaction may be present, but the core symptoms are defined more clearly than previously in the DSM-5 criteria. Because of concerns that individuals who may have met criteria for PDD not otherwise specified in the past may not meet ASD criteria, the DSM-5 criteria stipulated for the first time that a diagnosis may be established if the criteria were met in the past, meaning that diagnostic criteria may be met even if the behavioral manifestations of ASD do not appear currently but did appear in the past. Thus, people who received an ASD diagnosis according to the criteria of DSM-IV continue to receive the diagnosis under DSM-5.

Although the definitions of ASD have evolved over time, the core symptoms have remained largely the same. In the DSM-5,[25] social communication criteria are defined as (1) deficits in social-emotional reciprocity or the exchange of social behaviors, which include difficulties sharing enjoyment and interest with others, difficulties sustaining a back-and-forth in conversation, and reduced initiating and responding to social interaction; (2) deficits in using and understanding nonverbal communication; and (3) deficits in developing, understanding, and maintaining social relationships, which includes having interest in peers, understanding the nature of friendships and other common relationships, understanding social cues and norms, and sharing imaginative play with peers. Restricted, repetitive behaviors and fixated interests include (1) repetitive or stereotyped motor movements or use of objects (eg, lining up objects, repetitive interest in parts of objects), and/or speech (eg, echolalia, idiosyncratic speech); (2) insistence on sameness and difficulties with minor changes in routines or rigid patterns of verbal or nonverbal behavior; (3) fixated, narrow interests that are unusual in intensity (eg, perseverative interest in dinosaurs or anime) or focus (eg, strong attachment to or preoccupation with unusual objects); and (4) unusual responses to sensory aspects of the environment, including both unusual interest in and seeking of sensory input (eg, visual fascination with moving objects, excessive smelling or touching of objects) and being highly sensitive or aversive to sensory input (eg, unable to tolerate ordinary noises or textures).

Furthermore, diagnostic criteria in DSM-5 are accompanied by specifiers and modifiers. These provide a system to define "a more homogeneous subgrouping of individuals with the disorder who share certain features … ".[25] This information is expected to be relevant to service decisions for the individual. The system of specifiers for ASD includes a functional severity score across a 3-level scale (requiring support, requiring substantial support, requiring very substantial support), based on the impact of autism symptoms on everyday functioning. The severity scoring adds a dimensionality to the categorical diagnosis (**Fig. 1**). Thus, the specifiers, modifiers, and severity scores help characterize the ASD presentation in that particular individual. In addition, the specifiers and modifiers include information about accompanying intellectual disability; other neurodevelopmental, mental, behavioral, genetic and/or medical conditions; language impairment; and environmental factors. More than one specifier and modifier may be given, such as ASD without intellectual impairment with epilepsy. These changes were made to provide much-needed clarity given the heterogeneity of ASD.

The impairments associated with unusual social communication and interaction and restricted, repetitive, and unusual behaviors may be currently present or be reported as having occurred in the past, but the severity level for each domain is based on current behavior. In addition to meeting criteria in the 2 domains as described, symptoms must have been present in the early developmental period, although they may not express themselves fully until social demands exceed capacity levels, or may be masked by learned strategies, particularly later in life. These deficits must cause significant impairment, which impacts social, occupational, or other aspects of current functioning.

COMPREHENSIVE DIAGNOSTIC ASSESSMENTS

The goal of any diagnostic assessment is to obtain information that will be beneficial in decision making regarding the person being evaluated. This is achieved through a multidisciplinary assessment. Because ASD is a developmental disorder, an experienced developmental specialist should be on the team and, even more importantly, that developmental specialist must have specific and extensive expertise in

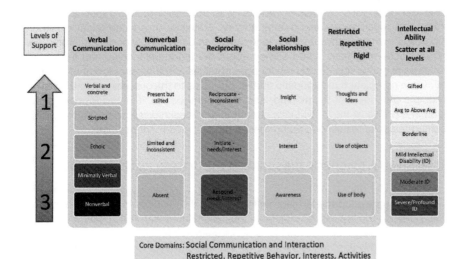

Fig. 1. Autism spectrum phenotype matrix. (*Courtesy of* C.E. Rice, PhD, Atlanta, GA.)

diagnosing and treating ASD. The consensus best-practice guidelines for diagnostic evaluation of ASD recommend a multidisciplinary evaluation that gathers information across multiple sources, including at a minimum direct observation of the child, a detailed parent interview for historical and current status, and direct assessment of developmental skills.[10,29–31] Recommendations include standardized assessment of the individual's development in cognitive, adaptive, and language skills regardless of the age at which the evaluation is conducted. Information obtained about the individual's behavior and functioning in natural settings, such as from educational or employment frameworks, complements the information gathered during the diagnostic assessment and can be very helpful in making the diagnosis. The multidisciplinary team typically consists of a psychologist, social worker, and speech and language pathologist, and when needed may also include occupational therapists, psychiatrists, developmental pediatricians, and neurologists. Additional information may be collected through the completion of questionnaires regarding the presence or absence of behaviors symptomatic of ASD, although there are some limitations regarding information obtained in questionnaires. However, the assessment of behavioral profiles, which is often accomplished through the use of questionnaires, can help with establishing co-occurring conditions or differential diagnoses, covered in the companion Cory Shulman and colleagues' article, "The Role of Diagnostic Instruments in Dual and Differential Diagnosis in Autism Spectrum Disorder (ASD) Across the Lifespan," in this issue.

The basic principles of comprehensive diagnostic assessment apply for all age groups. Assessment should be an ongoing, carefully designed multidisciplinary process, which captures the individual's functional, cognitive, intellectual, and language abilities, and behavioral profile. Individuals with ASD differ greatly from one another in terms of their cognitive skills, communication ability, interests, behaviors and social functioning, among other aspects, and the evaluation should allow professionals to appreciate strengths and weaknesses and to develop appropriate intervention strategies. In addition to individual differences at any given time point, developmental changes occur as each person with ASD grows and matures. Recommended best practices for ASD assessments include obtaining information regarding developmental, medical, and intervention history. When parents are unavailable, as is sometimes the case when evaluating adults, it is important to find other sources for information regarding developmental history. A sibling, or a close relative or friend who has known the individual for a long time, can often supply pertinent information, and a spouse may have heard stories about the individual's childhood from family members at gatherings. Screening for comorbidities and the assessment of other domains can complete the diagnostic profile. Additions to the process depend on the individual's age, level of functioning, and behavioral profile. The assessment should result in a profile of the individual's strengths and weaknesses, while clarifying diagnostic questions, resulting in recommendations for treatment planning.

ESTABLISHING A DIAGNOSIS THROUGHOUT THE LIFESPAN: DEVELOPMENTAL PERSPECTIVE

ASD is a neurodevelopmental disorder that affects the development of individuals over time. Because the behavioral manifestations associated with ASD change over time, the process of diagnosis and the instruments used to establish an accurate diagnosis must reflect a developmental perspective toward understanding behavior and ASD. The inconsistency in the presentation of autism symptomatology across settings, people, and levels of structure is particularly salient across development. At different ages there are different challenges to be addressed. For this reason, assessment strategies and instruments change as people with ASD move through the lifespan. The implementation of age-appropriate diagnostic assessment strategies is essential as a basis for understanding the individual's profile and establishing an intervention program.

For this review, ASD assessments have been divided into 4 developmental periods: infancy and toddlerhood (before 3 years), preschool (ages 3–6 years), school age (6–18 years including adolescence), and adulthood (over 18 years). This section examines the particular focus for each age group, in an attempt to characterize similarities and differences of ASD profiles at different ages. Typically for younger children the focus of the assessment is to answer the question "is this autism?", which is true for a first diagnosis at any age, although the presenting symptoms will be different for an initial diagnosis at different ages, as presented below. When summarizing the results of a diagnostic assessment, clinicians should be compassionate while presenting information and answering questions,[32] emphasizing that there are educational and treatment options available, providing parents with information about reliable Web sites and/or recommended books about ASD, as well as offering practical suggestions for handling pressing behavioral concerns. Assessments for school-aged children focus either on establishing an initial ASD diagnosis or on confirming an existing diagnosis, but parents are often interested in answering questions such as "what will my child be able to do?" and "why is my child doing so poorly at school when he or she is so smart?" During the elementary school years, an initial diagnostic assessment is usually for students with fluent verbal language and strong academic skills, often in math, science, and reading, who have been able to succeed academically despite possible difficulties with time management and organizational skills, as well as social interaction. These children may be diagnosed with ASD later as their academic skills may have "camouflaged" their autism symptoms.[33] This phenomenon may be one explanation why some girls are diagnosed later than their male counterparts. Similarly, diagnostic assessment in adulthood can also fall into the category of initial assessment, as the supports present in school are no longer present and more able adults with ASD begin to flounder socially and have trouble finding and sustaining employment.

As previously discussed, the ASD diagnostic evaluation is incomplete without additional information about other areas of assessment. Overall these may be referred to as skill assessment. Whereas, after the age of 2 years a diagnosis of ASD, made by experienced clinicians using standardized diagnostic tools and best clinical judgment, remains relatively stable, developmental skills vary over time. Children with ASD develop and learn new skills as they grow, just as children without ASD do, but the developmental trajectories of children with ASD are particularly variable. This instability has been attributed to children with ASD making marked progress later in development and to better cooperation during testing at later ages.[34–37] In general, IQ scores tend to remain stable or increase[38] and behavioral symptoms tend to decrease throughout childhood, adolescence, and even adulthood.[39,40]

Infancy and Toddlerhood

Even though the symptoms of ASD tend to appear early in development, the diagnosis of ASD cannot generally be reliably made until the age of 2 years. Research suggests that 80% to 90% of parents report their first concerns about their child's development by the child's second birthday and often well before.[41,42] Based on a systematic review of medical and educational records, 85% of children who eventually received a diagnosis of ASD had developmental concerns reported before 3 years, but only 40% to 45% of children received a comprehensive early diagnosis by age

3 years, and the median age of diagnosis is between age 4 and 5 years.[7] This gap between the time when concerns are first raised and the time of diagnosis is concerning. Several possible explanations for this disparity have been suggested. It may be that professionals and clinicians who see very young children are unaware of early markers of ASD; it is also possible that at such a young age, the expression of ASD symptoms overlaps with other syndromes or is still within typical development growth curves. It is imperative for clinicians of all disciplines to be vigilant for the early signs of ASD so that children can be effectively evaluated and efficiently diagnosed. Early evaluation shortens the time between symptom onset, diagnosis, and early intervention, which capitalizes on brain growth and neural plasticity that characterize early childhood and produces the most positive outcomes for children with ASD.[9,43–45] These early interventions are so crucial that the American Academy of Pediatrics is now recommending the initiation of interventions before the formal diagnosis of ASD, stating, "[a] definitive diagnosis is not necessary to institute services for documented delays that would be served through early intervention or school services".[46]

Before the age of 3 years, core symptoms of ASD include delays in language development for some children, aberrant social behavior, and poor play skills, particularly less doll play and more cause and effect play. At this age, skill assessment is typically based on observation of the child's use of materials during the assessment as well as on parental report. Accurate assessment requires engaging a child's attention and motivation to demonstrate his or her skills, which is particularly difficult for very young children.[47] When the demands become too difficult or the testing goes on too long behavior problems may emerge. It is important to distinguish whether the child's behavioral issues are a result of the testing context or of possible ASD. The developmental context of assessment of ASD in infants and toddlers requires the examination of the absence or delay of expected developmental milestones along with the emergence of autism symptomatology. Because toddlers who receive a diagnosis of ASD also typically exhibit developmental delays, it is necessary to rule out global developmental delay and/or language delays when diagnosing ASD in very young children. Specifically, it is important for clinicians to differentiate between delays and atypicalities in social engagement and reciprocity, as well as repetitive behaviors, due to overall cognitive delay or specific language impairment and those resulting from ASD. Although the absence of co-occurring cognitive and/or language delays at the time of first diagnosis is generally understood to be related to a more positive prognosis, the presence of marked delays does not necessarily predict that the toddler will have persisting cognitive and/or language impairment in later developmental periods.[48] Conversely, ASD may be overlooked in very young children or be dismissed as mild or transient.

Accumulating evidence from over a decade of prospective studies of at-risk siblings with an older sibling diagnosed with ASD reveals that the defining observable behavioral characteristics of ASD are not yet reliably discernible in infants 6 months and younger,[49,50] but emerge later.[11] Although a subset of children may in fact show symptoms in the first year of life, a more common pattern of symptom expression involves an early course of seemingly typical development or mild delays followed by the emergence of ASD-related atypical behaviors including atypical object exploration.[51–53] Another pattern of symptom onset in ASD suggests that some behaviors, such as eye contact and social smiling, may show a gradual decrease in frequency from 6 to 18 months, whereas others such as social vocalizations may fail to increase at the expected rate.[50] These findings suggest that various behaviors follow different developmental trajectories and occur during assorted developmental periods. Thus, because of the considerable clinical variation and etiologic heterogeneity, precise diagnosis of ASD in young children in the first year of life is difficult, as there is a subtle unfolding of social and communication difficulties alongside repetitive and restrictive behavior patterns.[54]

Despite the variability of behavioral manifestation of ASD in young children, particularly in the first year of life, research suggests that comprehensive, interdisciplinary assessment in the second year of life can lead to a reliable diagnosis of ASD.[55] Most children who receive an ASD diagnosis by the age of 2 years continue to receive that diagnosis at ages 3 to 4 years.[48,56–58] Factors associated with an earlier diagnosis include IQ within the range of intellectual disability, onset of developmental regression, and male sex.[40] Children from minority groups and lower socioeconomic status and girls typically receive a later diagnosis.[59]

Research suggests that the absence or delay in development of typical social behaviors is the best predictor of ASD in very young children.[60] This adds another level of complication to making the ASD diagnosis because one would be identifying the absence of appropriate developmental behaviors, such as *not* pointing to express interest in something, *not* responding to one's name when called, *not* showing social engagement, and *not* having normal eye contact. Other signs that are more easily identified, such as repetitive actions with objects, motor mannerisms, and sensory interests, also may be present in other disorders,[61] making them less reliable. Therefore, basing an ASD diagnosis on the presence of behaviors may not be as stable as the more difficult process of establishing a diagnosis based on reduced frequency or even complete absence of social behaviors. In addition, one must consider the variation in typical development at this stage of life, the protracted course of symptom emergence, the heterogeneity in the symptomatology, and the need to identify co-occurring conditions, discussed in the Cory Shulman and colleagues' article, "The Role of Diagnostic Instruments in Dual and Differential Diagnosis in Autism Spectrum Disorder (ASD) Across the Lifespan," in this issue.

Preschool Age (2–5 Years)

Between the ages of 2 and 3 years, ASD-related behaviors become more salient and diagnoses of ASD become highly stable.[57,62] At this age, many parents first notice that something is "not quite right" with their child's development. First concerns reported by parents in children this age often focus on communication and social areas, such as delays in language and decreased eye contact or decreased response to name, whereas others report nonautism-specific concerns such as motor delays, attention/hyperactivity concerns, or sleep problems.[63] The preschool years are a time of rapid developmental change, during which important communication, social, motor, play, and learning milestones are typically attained. Clinical presentation of young children with ASD is marked by high variability in the severity of ASD symptoms, heterogeneous language and cognitive abilities, and different behavioral profiles in the areas of attentional, behavioral, and emotional regulatory control problems.

There is growing clinical and research interest in conceptualizing ASD-related behaviors with regard to delays in skills that are observed in typical development as well as the presence of atypical behaviors.[64] Core symptoms of social communication in the preschool years are often characterized by deficits in joint attention (drawing another person's attention to an object or activity for the purpose of sharing interest), responding to their name or to a person speaking to them in a neutral tone, and/or initiating and maintaining physical social games, such as peekaboo or games involving motor imitation. Many children with ASD are not yet pointing to request (ie, proto-imperative) or to direct attention (ie, proto-declarative), or do so infrequently or in limited ways. Reduced eye contact remains a core feature throughout the lifespan, but in the preschool years children with ASD have reduced coordination of eye contact in highly motivating situations, such as requesting and sharing enjoyment. Children do not exhibit a variety of typical gestures[65] and do not use them to compensate for verbal language delays. Regarding peer interactions, young children may show a lack of interest in watching or approaching other children, or they may watch but not show interest in approaching or engaging. Responses to peer attempts at interaction may be inconsistent or rare. There may be delays in engaging in pretend play, including reduced imitative pretend play (eg, pretending to be a parent, pretending to cook/clean) or reduced imaginative and representational play.

Regarding repetitive behaviors, some of the earliest signs of ASD center on repetitive uses of objects, such as spinning or repetitive dropping or lining up of objects.[52] During early childhood repetitive motor behaviors are prevalent, and there is evidence that repetitive movements that involve the hands and fingers, such as finger splaying or hand posturing, are more predictive of ASD than repetitive whole-body movements.[66] Preschoolers who have some verbal language may show some repetitive or stereotyped speech, including immediate or delayed echolalia (repeating the speech of others), pronoun reversals (ie, confusing first- and second-person pronouns, saying "you" for "I"), or idiosyncratic language. Children who are not yet talking may engage in repetitive nonword vocalizations, such as unusual babbling or open-vowel sounds that appear to be self-stimulatory. In children who are not yet verbal it can be difficult to know whether an intense interest is present, and this may become clearer when a child is able to talk frequently about that interest. However, some young children with ASD will show unusual preoccupations or attachments to unusual objects, such as a strong interest in washing machines or clothes hangers. Insistence on sameness or difficulties with minor changes is less common than repetitive motor behaviors and uses of objects in young children but is still a common symptom, and more prevalent than in children with nonspectrum disabilities or with typical development.[61] Unusual sensory interests (seeking out visual, tactile, or other sensory input) are common in young children with ASD. Auditory sensory aversions, such as oversensitivity to ordinary but loud noises, occur at similar rates in children with and without ASD, but children with ASD more often experience tactile, visual, taste, or smell sensitivities than children with nonspectrum disorders or typical development.[61]

Symptom presentation and support needs of preschool children with ASD vary significantly, based on cognitive and language development and attentional and self-regulation skills. These factors seem to impact both current clinical presentation and trajectories of development. Longitudinal research has identified common trajectories in the development of children with ASD in preschool. A "severe, persistent" trajectory is characterized by a persistent, high level of social and repetitive behavior symptoms, with little progress in receptive and expressive language and nonverbal cognitive skills.[67,68] A moderate, stable group also has also been identified, characterized by moderate social communication deficits and repetitive behaviors, with below average and slightly increasing nonverbal cognitive skills.[68] Improving trajectories were also detected, in which children remained on the spectrum but showed improvement in social communication symptoms, language skills, and nonverbal IQ; results were mixed regarding whether restricted and repetitive behaviors improved.[67,68] These children also showed higher nonverbal cognitive skills at baseline than the moderate- and severe-persistent groups. Finally, a worsening trajectory was noted by Lord and colleagues,[67] characterized by worsening of social communication and repetitive behavior symptoms with little to no improvement in language or nonverbal cognitive skills.

Although social communication skills are more severely impacted in preschool children with significant language and cognitive delays, it seems that the presence of restricted and repetitive behaviors is relatively independent of developmental level in early childhood. Bishop and colleagues[69] found no significant relationship between restricted, repetitive behavior and nonverbal cognitive skills in children between 2 and 3 years, with the exception of sensory interests, where a higher percentage of children with moderate impairment in nonverbal IQ showed unusual sensory interests compared with children with nonverbal IQs over 70. However, after age 3 years, relationships do emerge between nonverbal IQ and several repetitive behaviors. A negative relationship with nonverbal IQ was observed for repetitive uses of objects, unusual sensory interests, hand and finger mannerisms, and complex/full-body mannerisms, and a positive relationship was seen for fixated interests and insistence on sameness[70,71]

In addition to assessment of autism symptoms, the above research illustrates the need for careful assessment of developmental skills in the preschool years to place ASD symptoms in the context of general developmental level and to plan for intervention needs. It may be beneficial to assess children multiple times over this time period to examine whether they have an improving or worsening trajectory to guide treatment focus and intensity. Furthermore, despite the relatively reliable stability of an ASD diagnosis established before the age of 3 years, research reveals a subset of children who receive an ASD diagnosis at age 3 years who were not previously identified, even though these high-risk siblings of children with an ASD diagnosis were seen for yearly assessment from age 6 months,[11,72] emphasizing the need for follow-up visits even if diagnostic criteria were not met at early assessments.

In the preschool years, co-occurring intellectual impairment and language delays are often a focus of evaluation and intervention. Although individual trajectories will vary, some evidence suggests that low IQ scores (IQ <70) at age 2 years have high stability into adulthood for children with ASD,[38] and this has implications for providing parents and professionals with guidance to plan proactively for intervention support needs. Many young children with ASD show an uneven profile of language development, in which receptive language is less developed compared with expressive language.[73] This pattern is unlike that of children with specific language impairment, who tend to have more marked deficits in language production than in comprehension.[74] The implication is that intervention programs for preschoolers with ASD should include an emphasis on facilitating their ability to understand language as well as working on their expressive language and communication skills.

School-Age Assessment Considerations (6–18 Years)

The developmental perspective of the DSM-5 ASD diagnostic criteria is often overlooked during the assessment process of school-age children. Individuals suspected of having ASD often have skill scatter within and across domains that can mask deficits. A diagnostic evaluation for ASD in school-age children can be an initial diagnosis, addressing the question "is this or is this not autism?", or a reevaluation addressing changes in ASD presentation as the child grows and the demands change. Those children who receive a later initial ASD diagnosis typically present with competing diagnoses,[75] making the diagnostic assessment complex, but necessary, as differential diagnosis and co-occurring conditions may inform treatment approaches and help with the consideration of long-term support needs (addressed in a Cory Shulman and colleagues' article, "The Role of Diagnostic Instruments in Dual and Differential Diagnosis in Autism Spectrum Disorder (ASD) Across the Lifespan," in this issue). Professionals assessing those students who undergo a reevaluation need to determine if an earlier ASD diagnosis is still the most descriptive of the student.

Complicating the diagnostic assessment is that school settings often reinforce academic achievement over social interactions. For example, an 8-year-old child who readily initiates and responds to social interactions with adults may not have insight into typical social relationships with peers. Assessments targeting social skills tend to rely on reports from others (ie, parents/legal guardians and teachers), with less information gathered directly from the student and/or peers. Even gold standard diagnostic assessments (ie, ADOS-2 and ADI-R) do not provide the opportunity to directly assess the individual interacting with other children of the same age. Current DSM-5 criteria for ASD require that deficits in all 3 social criteria be present,[25] one of which specifically deals with having peer relationships. Regardless of language and cognitive levels, social skill deficits continue to be the core impairment for students with ASD during the school years.[76] The school-age evaluation must include information about the student's unique areas of strengths and areas of need, and inform teachers regarding the most appropriate strategies to use to facilitate the child's learning. In particular, an ASD diagnosis indicates that the child will face significant challenges in attending to and learning socially mediated information.

Social-emotional reciprocity centers on the back-and-forth behaviors required to interact with others. Social impairments in a student increase during the school years and into adolescence due to the increasing complexity of social interactions as students mature. An awareness of social differences may become apparent and cause distress in students as they continue to struggle with peer-related social skills.[77] Inconsistencies in reciprocity often reflect differential and pragmatic initiating and responding, based on getting needs and wants addressed in the interaction. Difficulties in conversation and pragmatic use of language are included in this criterion. The focus of assessment of social-emotional reciprocity should be on whether the child is primed to attend, respond, and initiate when interacting. Assessments of language and cognitive skills are critical at this stage and should include an assessment of the student's social and pragmatic use of language,[78] including whether the student uses language to initiate and respond to social interactions with others; whether verbal language is being used to comment, show, and direct the attention of others; and whether verbalizations are used to gain items, information, or social attention. As children grow, nonverbal behaviors become more subtle and more frequent. Using a developmental framework, assessment should investigate an individual's use of eye contact and gestures, as well as use of body language and vocal tone, paying particular attention to whether these behaviors are limited or inappropriate and how well they are integrated into the social interaction.

Assessing deficits in development and maintenance of social relationships is probably the most difficult part of the evaluation in school-age children. Developmentally, youth move from having an awareness of others, to having an interest in others, to having insight into social relationships. At present, there are few protocols available for clinicians to use to assess this criterion. Gold standard assessments include few, if any, questions regarding these behaviors. For example, ADOS-2 does not directly assess peer interest or peer interaction because no peers are present.[67] The ADI-R contains 5 questions related to peer interactions,[79] but often parents do not know how their child interacts outside of the home. Determining a student's interest in interacting with peers is important, as lack of social interaction may not be a function of lack of interest in others but rather of a lack of skill.[80]

Wing and Gould[81] categorized children's interest in others as a way to help subtype subgroups of children with autism based on their social interactions with others. Children categorized with *social aloofness* displayed indifference toward social interactions. Some of these children may approach others to get items they want, but quickly return to being aloof once the item is obtained. Children who were labeled *passive* were those who did not spontaneously initiate social interactions with others but would accept the approaches of others. These children would also go when other children pulled them into their play but did not engage otherwise. Children who were described as *active but odd* made spontaneous initiations to both adults and other children, but this interaction was repetitive or idiosyncratic. These individuals did not have an interest in or feelings for others, nor did they modify their behavior based on social cues or social norms. Children whose social interactions were deemed *appropriate* for their mental age enjoyed social interaction for its own sake.

Another important aspect of school-age social functioning with peers lies within the "hidden curriculum",[82] which encompasses understanding implicit social messages. For example, does the student understand the unwritten social norms governing behavior of the student/school population that is not conducted in front of school personnel? This hidden curriculum can range from understanding which clothing should be worn to which students are popular and unpopular and why. Assessing students' ability to understand the hidden curriculum, particularly for students in middle and high school, is essential, because a lack of understanding in this area can cause social dysfunction.

Zablotsky and colleagues[83] found that 63% of individuals with ASD had been bullied at some point in their lifetime, and 38% had been bullied during the last 30 days. The individuals with ASD who were most often victims of bullying were children from lower socioeconomic backgrounds who attended public school. Middle school was a period of intensified bullying. Co-occurring conditions increased the likelihood of being bullied for students with ASD. Children with ASD in full inclusion, or who spent most their day in general education classrooms, were more likely to be bullied by peers than those children who were educated primarily in special education classrooms.[83]

Receiving an ASD diagnosis does not necessarily mean that the student will be eligible for autism educational services, because legislative mandates (Individuals with Disabilities Education Improvement Act [IDEA]) stipulate that eligibility for special education services depends on educational need.[84] Students with ASD and higher verbal and cognitive skill levels may not qualify if their academic achievement is not impacted. Comparison of recent CDC (Centers for Disease Control and Prevention) prevalence rates[7] and IDEA Child Count data from 2014 to 2015 indicates that educational eligibility is significantly lower than CDC rates.[85] This significant difference has been hypothesized to occur due to diagnostic substitution in the special education system, especially for students from racially and ethnically diverse backgrounds and for girls,[86] but this has not been proven. For whatever reason, the overall school-age population data confirms that a thorough assessment for ASD must take into account all areas of development and the presence of co-occurring conditions to best fit the student's educational needs and learning style.

Adulthood

As individuals with ASD transition into adulthood they leave behind many of the supports that they had within the educational system. With fewer supports and more demands for independence, many individuals with ASD struggle. Reassessment at this time may involve looking for public services and/or funds to provide the support that is no longer available through the school system. Some individuals with ASD may need supplemental income, supervision, supported living arrangements and employment, job training, medical care, help with transportation, and instruction in self-care and community living skills. There are also some individuals who will have attained adulthood without receiving an ASD diagnosis who will come for an initial

ASD diagnosis. Individuals whose first diagnostic assessment occurs in adulthood usually fall into 1 of 2 categories: those with severe intellectual and developmental impairments who are screened for ASD in institutional settings, and those with higher cognitive and adaptive functioning who are experiencing social deficits that could result from having ASD, which was not previously diagnosed. These latter individuals may self-refer for assessment because of employment-related difficulties or social interpersonal problems. This group of individuals is challenging diagnostically as their ASD may be subtle enough to go undetected until adulthood, may be complicated by other diagnoses that may be present and that overlap with ASD (eg, attention-deficit/hyperactivity disorder, anxiety), and/or may be present alongside other challenges that have developed as a result of living with unaddressed issues.

Referrals for a first diagnosis in adulthood are on the increase.[87–89] Unfortunately, consensus regarding the elements of a diagnosis in adulthood does not yet exist among professionals, resulting in ASD assessments based solely on observations and self-reporting, which are insufficient and can often be biased. Individuals coming for an ASD diagnosis for the first time as adults typically present challenging profiles. Some of them may have read about ASD, seen something in the media or been told by someone who knows them that they may have ASD. They have come to suspect that they may be "on the spectrum" after encountering information about ASD or after one of their children receives an ASD diagnosis. After perusing the Internet, they may decide that they indeed do have a profile appropriate for an ASD diagnosis and then refer themselves for an assessment, although they have already decided that they indeed meet ASD diagnostic criteria. For the professional who assesses them this presents a particular challenge. One 21 year old began his assessment by saying "Can we just assume I have ASD and continue the assessment with that conclusion?" Other adults have previously received diagnoses that may include intellectual disability, attention-deficit disorder, and various psychiatric disorders, such as social anxiety, depression, bipolar, and others. At some point, as these individuals reach adulthood, someone suggests that their issues are either better understood as characteristic of ASD (differential diagnosis) or that in addition to their other issues they also meet ASD diagnostic criteria (comorbid conditions). These adults present particularly complex diagnostic profiles and challenges for the examiner and the assessment challenges are addressed in a Cory Shulman and colleagues' article, "The Role of Diagnostic Instruments in Dual and Differential Diagnosis in Autism Spectrum Disorder (ASD) Across the Lifespan," in this issue. Understanding a person's early history and how their particular difficulties unfolded across childhood is extremely useful in differentiating ASD from other overlapping and co-occurring conditions, but this information sometimes is not available if a caregiver with a reliable memory of those early years is not available.

The National Institute for Health and Care Excellence (NICE) in the United Kingdom (https://www.nice.org.uk/guidance/cg142) has published recommendations for evaluations of ASD in adulthood, which are parallel to those for individuals with a suspicion of ASD at younger ages. At a minimum, NICE recommends assessment of core symptoms, early developmental history, behavior problems, functioning in employment and/or school and at home, as well as evaluation of current and past physical and mental disorders, other neurologic condition and hypersensitivities and hyposensitivities, and overattention to detail. This should all be done while considering clinical risks and contextual factors that could cause harm. NICE emphasizes the need to use standardized assessment tools whenever possible, particularly in complex cases. In cases of co-occurring psychiatric conditions it is important to include measures of mood disorders, anxiety, substance abuse, and other possible confounding factors. Therefore, the initial diagnosis of ASD in adulthood is complex because of the possible lack of developmental history and because of the likelihood of complicated histories involving other factors that may have disrupted development, such as abuse, neglect or trauma, or long-term mental health conditions. The inclusion of a sibling or spouse to provide information about earlier development can be helpful, if they are available and willing. Similarly, it becomes difficult to conclusively reach an initial ASD diagnosis in adulthood when there are other psychiatric and mental health concerns or when the individual has significant cognitive delay. Finally, when the individual is convinced that he or she has ASD before the completion of the assessment process, the results of the evaluation may not be valid.

SUMMARY OF DEVELOPMENTAL DIAGNOSTIC CONSIDERATIONS

In summary, a diagnostic evaluation of individuals with suspected ASD is impossible without having an understanding of their developmental profile at all ages. The diagnosis is dependent on understanding the developmental nature of the disorder, which requires the integration of information from many domains and the developmental context of that information. The profile of abilities and disabilities, strengths and weaknesses of the individual being assessed must inform the diagnosis, and more importantly inform intervention recommendations. The variability of the clinical presentation of ASD is striking and the ASD profile changes throughout the course of life. It is essential to thoroughly evaluate each individual's profile at various stages of development, particularly at pivotal transitions, such as receiving the diagnosis, entering/exiting school, and transitioning into adulthood. It is crucial to remember that the age of onset and the age of diagnosis are different. The earlier the diagnosis can be ascertained the better, but there are individuals who will not receive the diagnosis until adolescence or adulthood,[50] when social demands exceed capacities. There will also be individuals who have received other neurodevelopmental disorder diagnoses that no longer seem to address all their issues, and so the possibility of a diagnosis of ASD being more appropriate arises. Because the expression of ASD is heterogeneous and it manifests differently across the lifespan, clinicians must be experienced in typical developmental expectations, the expression of ASD at different ages, and other disorders (developmental or psychiatric), dependent on the age of the individual being assessed.

Research has shown that there are continuities and changes over time in the developmental trajectory of each individual with ASD. Therefore, generalizations about people with ASD must be tempered by the recognition that not all individuals with ASD conform to the common pattern and that the range of variation is great. With that caveat in mind, some of the common developmental patterns of lifetime development and change in ASD can be summarized. In most cases, an individual who has been given an authoritative diagnosis of ASD at one age will meet criteria for ASD at a later age,[57,90] although the symptom severity may change. Often severity is reduced. Rare cases of no to minimal symptom detection have been reported,[91] although in the great majority of cases autism cannot currently be "cured" nor does it spontaneously resolve itself. Intellectual and linguistic abilities also remain fairly consistent throughout early childhood, adolescence, and adulthood, and are implicated in long-term individual outcomes.[92] Thus, the intellectually able 5-year-old will likely do well in school and progress to higher education, employment, and independent living, whereas a child with ASD who is functioning like an 18-month-old at 5 years will most likely require special education and live and work in supported environments in adulthood. Some positive changes occur over time, with the diminution of the severity of autism symptoms and some of the difficult and challenging behaviors. Social skills continue to progress into adulthood. Some negative changes can also occur over time, with adolescence being a particularly vulnerable period for individuals growing up with ASD. Some may experience intellectual or behavior deterioration, which may be transient or a more permanent regression. For a minority of adolescents with ASD, epilepsy may occur for the first time. On the other hand, it is noteworthy that, for some individuals with ASD, adolescence is a period of improved social and intellectual functioning. Finally, as individuals transition into adulthood they often find themselves without the support they received within educational frameworks and the demands for financial and social functioning may be overwhelming, so that they need an updated ASD diagnosis to access services and get treatment that will help them manage to live as independently as possible.

DISCLOSURE

The authors have nothing to disclose.

REFERENCES

1. American Psychiatric Association. Diagnostic and statistical manual of mental disorders. 3rd edition. Washington, DC: Author; 1980.
2. American Psychiatric Association. Diagnostic and statistical manual of mental disorders. 3rd edition-revised. Washington, DC: Author; 1987.
3. Sinclair J. Being autistic together. Disabil Stud Q 2010;30(1). https://doi.org/10.18061/dsq.v30i1.1075.
4. Kanner L. Autistic disturbances of affective contact. Nervous Child 1943;2(3):217–50.
5. Asperger H. Die "autistischen psychopathen" im kindesalter. Eur Arch Psychiatry Clin Neurosci 1944;117(1):76–136.
6. Silberman S. Neurotribes: the legacy of autism and the future of neurodiversity. New York: Penguin; 2015.
7. Baio J, Wiggins L, Christensen DL, et al. Prevalence of autism spectrum disorder among children aged 8 years—autism and developmental disabilities monitoring network, 11 sites, United States, 2014. MMWR Surveill Summ 2018;67(6):1–23.
8. Fombonne E. The rising prevalence of autism. J Child Psychol Psychiatry 2018;59(7):717–20.
9. Dawson G, Jones EJ, Merkle K, et al. Early behavioral intervention is associated with normalized brain activity in young children with autism. J Am Acad Child Adolesc Psychiatry 2012;51:1150–9.
10. Huerta M, Lord C. Diagnostic evaluation of autism spectrum disorders. Pediatr Clin North Am 2012;59(1):103–11.
11. Zwaigenbaum L, Bauman ML, Stone WL, et al. Early identification of autism spectrum disorder: recommendations for practice and research. Pediatrics 2015;136(Supplement 1):S10–40.
12. Smith T, Klorman R, Mruzek DW. Predicting outcome of community-based early intensive behavioral intervention for children with autism. J Abnorm Child Psychol 2015;43(7):1271–82, 31.
13. Carr T, Lord C. A pilot study promoting participation of families with limited resources in early autism intervention. Res Autism Spectr Disord 2016;25:87–96.
14. Eisenberg L, Kanner L. Childhood schizophrenia: symposium, 1955: 6. Early infantile autism, 1943–55. Am J Orthopsychiatry 1956;26(3):556.

15. Waterhouse L. Autism overflows: increasing prevalence and proliferating theories. Neuropsychol Rev 2008;18(4):273–86.
16. Rimland B. Infantile autism. East Norwalk (CT): Appleton-Century-Crofts; 1964.
17. Rimland B. The differentiation of childhood psychoses: an analysis of checklists for 2,218 psychotic children. J Autism Child Schizophr 1971;1:161–74.
18. Wing L, Gould J. Systematic recording of behaviors and skills of retarded and psychotic children. J Autism Child Schizophr 1978;8(1):79–97.
19. Wing L. Language, social, and cognitive impairments in autism and severe mental retardation. J Autism Dev Disord 1981;11(1):31–44.
20. Ornitz EM. The modulation of sensory input and motor output in autistic children. J Autism Child Schizophr 1974;4(3):197–215.
21. Ornitz EM. Autism at the interface between sensory and information processing. In: Dawson G, editor. Autism: nature, diagnosis, and treatment. New York: Guilford Press; 1989. p. 174–207.
22. Rutter M. The development of infantile autism. Psychol Med 1974;4:147–63.
23. Prior MR. Cognitive abilities and disabilities in infantile autism: a review. J Abnorm Child Psychol 1979;7(4):357–80.
24. Ritvo ER, Freeman BJ. National Society for Autistic Children definition of the syndrome of autism. J Pediatr Psychol 1977;2(4):146–8.
25. American Psychiatric Association. Diagnostic and statistical manual of mental disorders. 5th edition. Washington, DC: Author; 2013.
26. Volkmar FR, Reichow B, Westphal A, et al. Autism and the autism spectrum: diagnostic concepts. In: Volkmar FR, Rogers S, Paul R, et al, editors. Handbook of autism and pervasive developmental disorders. 4th edition. Hoboken (NJ): John Wiley; 2014. p. 3–27.
27. American Psychiatric Association. Diagnostic and statistical manual of mental disorders. 4th edition. Washington, DC: Author; 1994.
28. American Psychiatric Association. Diagnostic and statistical manual of mental disorders. 4th edition. Washington, DC: Author; 2000.
29. Ozonoff S, Goodlin-Jones BL, Solomon M. Evidence-based assessment of autism spectrum disorders in children and adolescents. J Clin Child Adolesc Psychol 2005;34(3):523–40.
30. Esler AN, Ruble LA. DSM-5 diagnostic criteria for autism spectrum disorder with implications for school psychologists. Int J Sch Educ Psychol 2015;3(1):1–5.
31. Hammond RK, Campbell JM, Ruble LA. Considering identification and service provision for students with autism spectrum disorders within the context of response to intervention. Exceptionality 2013;21(1):34–50.
32. Hogan K, Marcus LM. From assessment to intervention. In: Goldstein S, Ozonoff S, editors. Assessment of autism spectrum disorder. New York: Guilford Publications; 2018. p. 318–38.
33. Lehnhardt FG, Falter CM, Gawronski A, et al. Sex-related cognitive profile in autism spectrum disorders diagnosed late in life: implications for the female autistic phenotype. J Autism Dev Disord 2016;46(1):139–54.
34. Charman T, Taylor E, Drew A, et al. Outcome at 7 years of children diagnosed with autism at age 2: predictive validity of assessments conducted at 2 and 3 years of age and pattern of symptom change over time. J Child Psychol Psychiatry 2005; 46(5):500–13.
35. Moore V, Goodson S. How well does early diagnosis of autism stand the test of time? Follow-up study of children assessed for autism at age 2 and development of an early diagnostic service. Autism 2003;7(1):47–63.

36. Rapin I, Dunn M. Update on the language disorders of individuals on the autistic spectrum. Brain Dev 2003;25(3):166–72.
37. Turner LM, Stone WL, Pozdol SL, et al. Follow-up of children with autism spectrum disorders from age 2 to age 9. Autism 2006;10(3):243–65.
38. Anderson DK, Liang JW, Lord C. Predicting young adult outcome among more and less cognitively able individuals with autism spectrum disorders. J Child Psychol Psychiatry 2014;55(5):485–94.
39. Howlin P, Moss P, Savage S, et al. Social outcomes in mid-to later adulthood among individuals diagnosed with autism and average nonverbal IQ as children. J Am Acad Child Adolesc Psychiatry 2013;52(6):572–81.
40. Shattuck PT, Durkin M, Maenner M, et al. Timing of identification among children with an autism spectrum disorder: findings from a population-based surveillance study. J Am Acad Child Adolesc Psychiatry 2009;48(5):474–83.
41. Chawarska K, Klin A, Paul R, et al. A prospective study of toddlers with ASD: short-term diagnostic and cognitive outcomes. J Child Psychol Psychiatry 2009;50(10):1235–45.
42. Howlin P, Moore A. Diagnosis in autism: a survey of over 1200 patients in the UK. Autism 1997;1(2):135–62.
43. Courchesne E, Mouton PR, Calhoun ME, et al. Neuron number and size in prefrontal cortex of children with autism. JAMA 2011;306(18):2001–10.
44. Dawson G, Rogers SJ, Munson J, et al. Randomized, controlled trial of an intervention for toddlers with autism: the early start Denver model. Pediatrics 2010; 125:17–23.
45. Koegel LK, Koegel RL, Ashbaugh K, et al. The importance of early identification and intervention for children with or at risk for autism spectrum disorders. Int J Speech Lang Pathol 2014;16(1):50–6.
46. Hyman SL, Levy SE, Myers SM. Identification, evaluation, and management of children with autism spectrum disorder. Pediatrics 2019;145(1) [pii:e20193447].
47. Ozonoff SE, Rogers SJ, Hendren RL. Autism spectrum disorders: a research review for practitioners. Washington, DC: American Psychiatric Association Publishing; 2003.
48. Kim SH, Macari S, Koller J, et al. Examining the phenotypic heterogeneity of early autism spectrum disorder: subtypes and short-term outcomes. J Child Psychol Psychiatry 2016;57(1):93–102.
49. Bryson SE, Zwaigenbaum L, Brian J, et al. A prospective case series of high-risk infants who developed autism. J Autism Dev Disord 2007;37(1):12–24.
50. Ozonoff S, Iosif AM, Baguio F, et al. A prospective study of the emergence of early behavioral signs of autism. J Am Acad Child Adolesc Psychiatry 2010; 49(3):256–66.
51. Kim SH, Lord C. Combining information from multiple sources for the diagnosis of autism spectrum disorders for toddlers and young preschoolers from 12 to 47 months of age. J Child Psychol Psychiatry 2012;53(2):143–51.
52. Ozonoff S, Macari S, Young GS, et al. Atypical object exploration at 12 months of age is associated with autism in a prospective sample. Autism 2008;12(5): 457–72.
53. Paul R, Fuerst Y, Ramsay G, et al. Out of the mouths of babes: vocal production in infant siblings of children with ASD. J Child Psychol Psychiatry 2011;52(5): 588–98.
54. Wing L, Gould J, Gillberg C. Autism spectrum disorders in the DSM-V: better or worse than the DSM-IV? Res Dev Disabil 2011;32(2):768–73.

55. Esler AN, Bal VH, Guthrie W, et al. The autism diagnostic observation schedule, toddler module: standardized severity scores. J Autism Dev Disord 2015;45(9): 2704–20.
56. Guthrie W, Swineford LB, Nottke C, et al. Early diagnosis of autism spectrum disorder: stability and change in clinical diagnosis and symptom presentation. J Child Psychol Psychiatry 2013;54(5):582–90.
57. Lord C, Risi S, DiLavore PS, et al. Autism from 2 to 9 years of age. Arch Gen Psychiatry 2006;63(6):694–701.
58. Chawarska K, Klin A, Paul R, et al. Autism spectrum disorder in the second year: stability and change in syndrome expression. J Child Psychol Psychiatry 2007; 48(2):128–38.
59. Thomas KC, Ellis AR, McLaurin C, et al. Access to care for autism-related services. J Autism Dev Disord 2007;37(10):1902–12.
60. Barton ML, Dumont-Mathieu T, Fein D. Screening young children for autism spectrum disorders in primary practice. J Autism Dev Disord 2012;42(6):1165–74.
61. Richler J, Bishop SL, Kleinke JR, et al. Restricted and repetitive behaviors in young children with autism spectrum disorders. J Autism Dev Disord 2007; 37(1):73–85.
62. Guthrie W, Swineford LB, Wetherby AM, et al. Comparison of DSM-IV and DSM-5 factor structure models for toddlers with autism spectrum disorder. J Am Acad Child Adolesc Psychiatry 2013;52(8):797–805.
63. Guinchat V, Chamak B, Bonniau B, et al. Very early signs of autism reported by parents include many concerns not specific to autism criteria. Res Autism Spectr Disord 2012;6(2):589–601.
64. Foss-Feig JH, McPartland JC, Anticevic A, et al. Re-conceptualizing ASD within a dimensional framework: positive, negative, and cognitive feature clusters. J Autism Dev Disord 2016;46(1):342–51.
65. Wetherby AM, Watt N, Morgan L, et al. Social communication profiles of children with autism spectrum disorders late in the second year of life. J Autism Dev Disord 2007;37(5):960–75.
66. Luyster R, Gotham K, Guthrie W, et al. The autism diagnostic observation schedule—toddler module: a new module of a standardized diagnostic measure for autism spectrum disorders. J Autism Dev Disord 2009;39(9):1305–20.
67. Lord C, Luyster R, Guthrie W, et al. Patterns of developmental trajectories in toddlers with autism spectrum disorder. J Consult Clin Psychol 2012;80(3):477.
68. Visser JC, Rommelse NN, Lappenschaar M, et al. Variation in the early trajectories of autism symptoms is related to the development of language, cognition, and behavior problems. J Am Acad Child Adolesc Psychiatry 2017;56(8):659–68.
69. Bishop SL, Richler J, Lord C. Association between restricted and repetitive behaviors and nonverbal IQ in children with autism spectrum disorders. Child Neuropsychol 2006;12(4–5):247–67.
70. Bishop SL, Hus V, Duncan A, et al. Subcategories of restricted and repetitive behaviors in children with autism spectrum disorders. J Autism Dev Disord 2013; 43(6):1287–97.
71. Kim SH, Thurm A, Shumway S, et al. Multisite study of new autism diagnostic interview-revised (ADI-R) algorithms for toddlers and young preschoolers. J Autism Dev Disord 2013;43(7):1527–38.
72. Ozonoff S, Young GS, Landa RJ, et al. Diagnostic stability in young children at risk for autism spectrum disorder: a baby siblings research consortium study. J Child Psychol Psychiatry 2015;56(9):988–98.

73. Ellis Weismer S, Lord C, Esler A. Early language patterns of toddlers on the autism spectrum compared to toddlers with developmental delay. J Autism Dev Disord 2010;40(10):1259–73.

74. Laws G, Bishop DV. A comparison of language abilities in adolescents with Down syndrome and children with specific language impairment. J Speech Lang Hear Res 2003;46(6):1324–39.

75. Simonoff E, Pickles A, Charman T, et al. Psychiatric disorders in children with autism spectrum disorders: prevalence, co-morbidity, and associated factors in a population-derived sample. J Am Acad Child Adolesc Psychiatry 2008;47(8):921–9.

76. Carter AS, Davis NO, Klin A, et al. Social development in autism. In: Volkmar FR, Paul R, Klin A, et al, editors. Handbook of autism and pervasive developmental disorders: diagnosis, development, neurobiology, and behavior, vol. 1. Hoboken (NJ): John Wiley & Sons; 2005.

77. Tantam D. The challenge of adolescents and adults with Asperger syndrome. Child Adolesc Psychiatr Clin N Am 2003;12:143–63.

78. Philofsky A, Fidler DJ, Heburn S. Pragmatic language profiles of school-age children with autism spectrum disorder and Williams syndrome. Am J Speech Lang Pathol 2007;16(4):368–80.

79. Rutter M, Le Couteur A, Lord C. Autism diagnostic interview-revised, vol. 29. Los Angeles (CA): Western Psychological Services; 2003. p. 30.

80. White SW, Koening K, Scahill L. Social skills development in children with autism spectrum disorder: a review of intervention research. J Autism Dev Disord 2007;37(10):1858–68.

81. Wing L, Gould J. Severe impairments of social interaction and associated abnormalities in children: epidemiology and classification. J Autism Dev Disord 1979;9(1):11–29.

82. Lee HJ. Cultural factors related to the hidden curriculum for students with autism and related disabilities. Interv Sch Clin 2011;46(3):141–9.

83. Zablotsky B, Bradshaw CP, Anderson CM, et al. Risk factors for bullying among children with autism spectrum disorders. Autism 2014;18:419–27.

84. Sullivan AL. School-based autism identification: prevalence, racial disparities, and systematic correlates. Sch Psychol Rev 2015;42:298–316.

85. Barnard-Brak L. Brief Report: educational versus clinical diagnoses of autism spectrum disorder: updated and expanded findings. Sch Psychol Rev 2019;48(2):185–9.

86. Bent CA, Barbaro J, Dissanayake C. Change in autism diagnoses prior to and following the introduction of DSM-5. J Autism Dev Disord 2017;47(1):163–71.

87. Stuart-Hamilton I, Morgan H. What happens to people with autism spectrum disorders in middle age and beyond? Report of a preliminary on-line study. Adv Ment Health Intellect Disabil 2011;5(2):22–8.

88. Mukaetova-Ladinska EB, Perry E, Baron M, et al, Autism Ageing Writing Group. Ageing in people with autistic spectrum disorder. Int J Geriatr Psychiatry 2012;27(2):109–18.

89. Povey C, Mills R, Gomez de la Cuesta G. Autism and ageing: issues for the future. Clin Pract 2011;230–2.

90. Howlin P. Outcomes in autism spectrum disorders. In: Volkmar FR, Paul R, Klin A, et al, editors. Handbook of autism and pervasive developmental disorders: diagnosis, development, neurobiology, and behavior, vol. 1, 3rd edition. Hoboken (NJ): John Wiley & Sons; 2005. p. 201–20.

91. Fein D, Barton M, Eigsti IM, et al. Optimal outcome in individuals with a history of autism. J Child Psychol Psychiatry 2013;54(2):195–205.

92. Lord C, Corsello C, Grzadzinski R. Diagnostic instruments in autism spectrum disorders. In: Volkmar FR, Rogers S, Paul R, et al, editors. Handbook of autism and pervasive developmental disorders. 4th edition. Hoboken (NJ): John Wiley; 2014. p. 609–60.

The Role of Diagnostic Instruments in Dual and Differential Diagnosis in Autism Spectrum Disorder Across the Lifespan

Cory Shulman, PhD[a],*, Catherine E. Rice, PhD[b],
Michael J. Morrier, PhD[b], Amy Esler, PhD[c]

KEYWORDS

- Autism • Dual diagnosis • Differential diagnosis • Co-occurring conditions
- Lifespan • Diagnostic instruments

KEY POINTS

- The heterogeneity inherent in autism spectrum disorder (ASD) makes the identification and diagnosis of ASD complex.
- This is particularly true as ASD heterogeneity presents differently over time.
- The results of a diagnostic assessment is only as good as the instruments used in the assessment and the professional expertise of the practitioner.
- A call to action is necessary for meeting the diagnostic challenges of ASD to improve the diagnostic process and to help understand each individual's particular ASD profile.

BACKGROUND

Specifying autism spectrum disorder (ASD) has been the goal of clinicians and researchers alike over the past 40 years, in an attempt to understand the heterogeneity and the chronogeneity[1] in autism. Chronogeneity refers to the study of the heterogeneity of autism in relationship to the dimension of time, which is not always captured in the assessment process. Autism is a label used to describe a constellation of behaviorally identified criteria that cluster together in diverse ways and differing severities to form a definable pattern in a person's developmental progression, and its utility lies in

[a] The Paul Baerwald School of Social Work and Social Welfare, The Hebrew University of Jerusalem, Mount Scopus, Jerusalem, 91905, Israel; [b] Emory Autism Center, 1551 Shoup Court, Department of Psychiatry & Behavioral Sciences, Emory University School of Medicine, Decatur, GA 30033, USA; [c] Division of Clinical Behavioral Neuroscience, Department of Pediatrics, University of Minnesota 2540 Riverside Ave S., RPB 550, Minneapolis, MN 55454, USA
* Corresponding author.
E-mail address: cory.shulman@mail.huji.ac.il

Child Adolesc Psychiatric Clin N Am 29 (2020) 275–299
https://doi.org/10.1016/j.chc.2020.01.002
1056-4993/20/© 2020 Elsevier Inc. All rights reserved.

Abbreviations	
ADHD	Attention-deficit/hyperactivity disorder
ADI-R	Autism diagnostic interview–revised
ADOS-2	Autism diagnostic observation schedule, second edition
ASD	Autism spectrum disorder
ASEBA	Achenbach system of empirically based assessment
CARS-2	Childhood autism rating scale, second edition
GAD	Generalized anxiety disorder
ID	Intellectual disability

describing and predicting behavior that does not fit the typical progression. The autism diagnosis reflects criteria that specify the phenomenological characteristics of autism, that is, the presence or absence of those behaviors which define it. Throughout the 70 years since it was first defined as a diagnostic entity,[2] autism as a diagnosis has retained its features of deficits in social interaction and social communication, as well as the presence of restricted interests and repetitive behaviors. Social interaction deficits specific to autism focus on reduced social interest and social motivation, decreased reciprocity in social engagement, limited understanding and use of nonverbal communication, and deficits in understanding social relationships and social cues. Restricted and repetitive behaviors include unusual preoccupations, repetitive play behaviors, repetitive motor movements and speech, and insistence on following nonfunctional routines and rituals.

Although the definitions of ASD have evolved over time, the core symptoms have remained largely the same. In the *Diagnostic and Statistical Manual of Mental Disorders, Fifth Edition (DSM-5)*,[3] social communication criteria are defined as: (1) deficits in social-emotional reciprocity or the exchange of social behaviors, which include difficulties sharing enjoyment and interest with others, difficulties sustaining a back-and-forth in conversation, and reduced initiating and responding to social interaction; (2) deficits in using and understanding nonverbal communication; and (3) deficits in developing, understanding, and maintaining social relationships, which includes having interest in peers, understanding the nature of friendships and other common relationships, understanding social cues and norms, and sharing imaginative play with peers. Restricted, repetitive behaviors and fixated interests include: (1) repetitive or stereotyped motor movements, use of objects (eg, lining, repetitive interest in parts of objects), and/or speech (eg, echolalia, idiosyncratic speech); (2) insistence on sameness and difficulties with minor changes in routines or rigid patterns of verbal or nonverbal behavior; (3) fixated, narrow interests that are unusual in intensity (eg, perseverative interest in dinosaurs or anime) or focus (eg, strong attachment to or preoccupation with unusual objects); and (4) unusual responses to sensory aspects of the environment, including both unusual interest in and seeking of sensory input (eg, visual fascination with moving objects, excessive smelling or touching of objects) and being highly sensitive or aversive to sensory input (eg, unable to tolerate ordinary noises or textures).

The heterogeneity and chronogeneity (heterogeneity over time) of autism relate to an individual's personal trajectory, which must be understood to adapt treatments at any given time. This is particularly crucial as individuals initially diagnosed in childhood reach adulthood, and then once again the purpose, meaning, and function of an ASD diagnosis must be examined. Alongside the aging population of individuals with ASD,[4,5] a cohort of younger children is being identified and developmental trajectories from infancy and toddlerhood allow a deeper understanding of changing profiles of ASD at different ages. The complexity involved in considering not simply the core symptomatology of ASD but also co-occurring conditions and causes has been incorporated into the *DSM-5* criteria for ASD as specifiers and modifiers, which provide a system to define "a more homogeneous subgrouping of individuals with the disorder who share certain features...".[3] The system of specifiers for ASD includes a functional severity score across a 3-level scale (requiring support, requiring substantial support, and requiring very substantial support), based on adaptive functioning. The severity scoring adds a dimensionality to the categorical diagnosis and can help in treatment decisions. No longer is it enough to diagnose a person with ASD; it is necessary to address specifiers, modifiers, and severity scores to help indicate how ASD presents in that particular individual. In addition, the specifiers and modifiers include information about accompanying intellectual disability (ID); other neurodevelopmental, mental, behavioral, genetic, and/or medical conditions; language impairment; and environmental factors. More than 1 specifier and modifier may be given, such as ASD without intellectual impairment with epilepsy. After discussing the components of a comprehensive assessment in the Cory Shulman and colleagues' article, "Diagnosis of Autism Spectrum Disorder (ASD) Across the Lifespan," in this issue, this article deals with the diagnostic differentials that come into play and how the correct choice of tests can help in understanding the individual ASD profile. Several disorders can be mistaken for ASD because of atypical patterns of social communication and/or odd behaviors. Moreover, symptoms of other disorders can appear in individuals with ASD. The presence of one or more co-occurring conditions is also referred to as comorbidity and is quite common in ASD; therefore, it is critical that diagnosticians understand the areas of overlap and how to understand ASD manifestations as well as other related conditions. Developmental stages including early childhood (up to age 3 years); preschool (ages 3–5 years); elementary school (ages 6–18 years); and adulthood (18 years and beyond) provide the perspective for understanding the choice of instruments and the co-occurring conditions to be considered.

DIAGNOSTIC INSTRUMENTS IN THE AUTISM SPECTRUM DISORDER DIAGNOSTIC BATTERY

The instruments used to establish the diagnosis are the central component of the diagnostic evaluation, as they are the conduit of pertinent information regarding the individual being assessed and the method of measurement. It is important to carefully choose the correct instruments to avoid mismeasurement and/or misinformation, recognizing that different tools can be used at various ages and levels of functioning, providing different types of information. Some of the specific challenges encountered when deciding which instruments to use arise from changes in and broadening of the ASD diagnostic criteria, the diverse manifestations of ASD at different ages, and the need for differential and dual diagnoses. Although the universal goal of assessing ASD is obtaining information that will in some way benefit each individual and his or her family, the specific focus and tools for assessment of ASD vary markedly, depending on the age of the person being assessed. Since many assessments for ASD take place through local developmental clinics or agencies, or public schools, it is particularly important to understand which assessment tools are appropriate for which levels of functioning and for which ages.[6] Good choices regarding correct assessment tools for diagnosis, paired with training and experience in ASD and other neurodevelopmental disorders, make it possible for clinicians in a variety of settings to perform meaningful, professional evaluations for individuals across the age range.[7-9] The next 2 sections deal with issues involved in the selection of diagnostic instruments and present an overview of existing instruments. Instruments are included in the survey only if there is at least 1 empirical article reporting reliability and validity that was not conducted by the authors of the instrument.

Psychometric Issues in Autism Spectrum Disorder Diagnostic Instruments

The diagnosis of ASD is impacted by the clinician's experience and skill in identifying characteristics of ASD and other typical and atypical presentations and by the instruments used to measure these behaviors. In particular, assessment tools directly influence the manner in which the disorder is defined and understood. The choice of instruments used for diagnostic ascertainment depends on a number of considerations. Foremost, the instrument should be standardized, maximizing both sensitivity and specificity while remaining reliable and valid. The instrument should be appropriate for the age and ability level of the individual and should capture the variety of autistic symptoms being presented. Better instruments yield more accurate, reliable, and valid information, and ultimately inform both researchers and clinicians. Over the past 30 years, many instruments have been developed for use in establishing an ASD diagnosis across the lifespan. The reliability of any test or scale is critical for clinical practice as well as for research. Reliability refers to the degree of accuracy of the scores obtained from the instrument. Validity is defined as the degree to which empirical evidence supports an interpretation of the scores as representing the construct being assessed. Understanding the psychometrics of assessments and the constraints on their use can help in deciding which test to use for each individual. The reliability and validity of the instruments are presented in **Table 1**.

Specific Autism Spectrum Disorder Diagnostic Instruments

The Autism Diagnostic Observation Schedule, second edition (ADOS-2[38–40]), is a semi-structured assessment of communication, social interaction, restrictive and repetitive behaviors, and play in younger children and imagination in adolescents and adults. The appropriate module of the 5 in the schedule is chosen according to the individual's age and expressive language ability. Each module takes between 45 and 60 minutes to administer, and because the individual's developmental and speech level is taken into account in choosing the correct module, the issues that arise during the assessment are not the result of developmental delay or language and speech limitations. Each module consists of a variety of structured and unstructured activities that are designed to elicit the social communication and repetitive behavior symptoms of ASD relevant to the language level and age appropriate to that module. Generally, modules designed for children with less language include activities with opportunities for toy play, requesting continuation of examiner-led activities, pretend play, and social games, and for those with phrase speech, having a conversation and talking about a picture and a book together. Modules designed for children and adults with complex sentences include structured activities to elicit information on the participant's descriptive language, the ability to retell events, conversational skills, and imaginative/creative play or use of materials. These modules also ask direct questions, in a conversational style, designed to assess the participant's insight into emotions, relationships, and common social situations (eg, bullying, getting along with others[41–44]).

Examiners take notes during the ADOS-2 administration and the codes are rated immediately after administration. Guidelines are provided for deciding on the rating for each code and algorithms are provided for formulating ADOS-2 classifications, which are used along with all additional information collected during the assessment to decide on a diagnosis using best clinical judgment. The ADOS-2 scores can be

Table 1
Psychometric properties of autism spectrum disorder screening tools and questionnaires

Measure	Intended Students	Administration	Sensitivity/Specificity
M-CHAT-R/F[10]	16–30 mo, any verbal or cognitive level	Parent/caregiver checklist Follow-up interview is recommended for children who fail	*ASD vs NS, with follow-up interview:* Se = 0.97, Sp = 0.99[10] *ASD vs NS, checklist alone:* Failing 2 critical items: Se = 0.70, Sp = 0.38[11] Se = 0.77, Sp = 0.43[12] Failing any 3 items: Se = 0.92, Sp = 0.27[12] Se = 0.88, Sp = 0.38[11] Failing either cutoff: Se = 0.60, Sp = 0.50[13]
GARS/GARS-2	3–22 y, any verbal or cognitive level	Parent/caregiver or teacher questionnaire (5–10 min); Structured parent interview form (unscored) for information about development during early childhood	*ASD vs NS:* Se = 0.83, Sp = 0.68[12] Se = 0.53, Sp = 0.54[14] *ASD only:* Se = 0.38[15]
SCQ	4 + years; nvma ≥2 y	Parent/caregiver questionnaire (10 min) Lifetime Version: Coverage of past and current symptoms Current version current symptoms only	*ASD vs NS:* Se = 0.85, Sp = 0.75[16,17] Se = 0.88, Sp = 0.72[18,19] Se = 0.86, Sp = 0.78[20–22] Se = 0.71, Sp = 0.71[23] Se = 0.74, Sp = 0.54[12] Se: 0.92, Sp = 0.62[24–27] *AUT vs NS:* Se = 0.96, Sp = 0.80[16] Se = 0.78, Sp = 0.71[23]

(continued on next page)

Table 1
(continued)

Measure	Intended Students	Administration	Sensitivity/Specificity
SRS-2	4–18 y, any verbal or cognitive level	Parent/caregiver or teacher questionnaire (15–20 min)	*ASD vs NS:* Se = 0.78, Sp = 0.67[20] Se = 0.75, Sp = 0.96[28] Se = 0.92, Sp = 0.08 *(parent ratings)*[29] Se = 0.84, Sp = 0.41 *(teacher ratings)*[29] Se = 0.76, Sp = 0.82[30]
ASRS	Age 2–18 y	Parent/caregiver or teacher questionnaire	*ASD vs NS* *DSM-IV score:* Se = 0.91, Sp = 0.92[31–34] *Total score:* Se = 0.90, Sp = 0.92[31] *Total score:* Se = 0.94, Sp = 0.84[35,36] *DSM-5:* Se = 0.91, Sp = 0.16[37] *Total score:* Se = 0.83, Sp = 0.24[37]

Abbreviations: AUT, autistic disorder; GARS/GARS-2, Gilliam Autism Rating Scale; ID, intellectual disability; M-CHAT–R/F, Modified Checklist for Autism in Toddlers–Revised, with Follow-up Interview; NS, nonspectrum; nvma, nonverbal mental age; SCQ, Social Communication Questionnaire; Se, sensitivity; Sp, specificity; SRS-2, social responsiveness scale, second edition.

mapped onto the *DSM-5* diagnostic criteria for ASD. Reliability was calculated for each module separately and mean agreement scores range from 78% to 98%, and when data were collapsed across all modules the interclass correlations coefficient for the social affect domain was 0.96, whereas the restrictive and repetitive behavior coefficient was 0.84. Validity ratings for sensitivity and specificity of the ADOS-2 range from 83% to 91% (sensitivity) and from 86% to 94% (specificity) over all the modules. Thus, the psychometrics of the ADOS-2 are quite robust and reflect an instrument that is both reliable and valid for diagnostic assessment over the lifespan.

The Autism Diagnostic Interview–Revised (ADI-R[45]) is an extended, semi-structured interview of a parent or caregiver who is knowledgeable about the individual's behavior, development, and functioning currently and in the past, focusing on the period from 4 to 5 years of age. It is administered by an experienced clinician and produces information needed to diagnose ASD, as well as characterizing current behavior patterns. It consists of 93 questions focusing primarily on history, language and communication, reciprocal social interactions, and restricted and repetitive behaviors, including preoccupations and interests. The assessed individual must have a mental age of at least 2 years. The interview takes approximately 1.5 to 3 hours to complete. The interviewer records and codes detailed responses of the informant using the interview protocol. After the protocol is coded, the codes are transferred to the appropriate algorithm according to the purpose of the interview. There are 2 algorithms to be used for different purposes: (1) a diagnostic algorithm for establishing an ASD diagnosis and (2) a current behavior algorithm for characterizing present behavior patterns. Diagnostic algorithms take reports of behaviors historically, focusing on the period of time between 4 and 5 years of age except for those items that are coded if the behavior "ever" appeared.

The diagnostic algorithm generates either a classification of autism, indicating the informants described behaviors consistent with those seen in ASD, or a classification of nonspectrum, indicating the informants did not describe a pattern of behavior or development that met the threshold for ASD. Summary scores for 4 domains (ie, qualitative abnormalities in reciprocal social interactions, qualitative abnormalities in communication, restricted and repetitive behaviors, and whether the behaviors were present before the age of 36 months) are compared with the diagnostic cutoffs to determine the presence of ASD. The algorithm for current behavior reflects symptoms at the time of the interview and can be used for treatment plans; it does not generate a classification. Interrater and test-retest reliability and validity data are presented in the manual. With its high sensitivity and specificity, the ADI-R is a necessary part of an ASD diagnostic assessment, as it collects information about the individual from the informant in a comprehensive manner, resulting in an ability to integrate information from the individual's past and present.

The Childhood Autism Rating Scale, Second Edition (CARS-2[46]) comprises 3 forms. The CARS-2 standard form is for ages 6 years and younger with an estimated IQ of 79 or lower. The second form, the CARS-2 high functioning version, is designed for those 6 and older with an estimated IQ of 80 or higher. There is also a CARS-2 questionnaire for parents or caregivers, which is designed to assist in gathering information regarding behaviors related to ASD to help inform scoring of the other 2 versions. Each version of the CARS-2 consists of 15 items associated with the diagnosis of ASD. The CARS-2 helps to identify individuals with ASD, to evaluate the degree of severity of the disorder, and to help determine whether a more comprehensive evaluation for ASD is warranted. The CARS-2 can differentiate children with and without ASD as well as children with ASD from children with other developmental disorders, particularly those with moderate to severe ID. The ratings of the CARS-2 are based on the clinician's observations, which are rated on a scale of 1 (within normal limits), 2 (mildly abnormal), 3 (moderately abnormal), and 4 (severely abnormal). Item scores for CARS-2 are summed and categorized according to cutoff scores, with any score under 30 indicating non-ASD; 30 to 36.5 is considered mild to moderate ASD; 37 to 60 is considered severe ASD.

Diagnostic Screeners and Rating Scales

Questionnaires are often added to the diagnostic battery to focus on particular aspects of behaviors or to provide additional information that can complement or confirm information already collected. Questionnaires, such as all diagnostic tools, must be reliable, valid, and have high sensitivity (finding cases of ASD) and specificity (finding only cases of ASD). Many ASD questionnaires are in use today, some of which are used as screeners and some of which are used for diagnostic purposes, but all questionnaires are completed by the individual being assessed or by an informant, such as a parent or caregiver who knows the individual well. Self- and informant-reporting are influenced by previous knowledge and the reasons for seeking a diagnosis. Behaviors are seen by some informants as indicative of ASD and will be reported as such, whereas others (eg, parents) describing the same behavior in their child will not relate to the behavior as symptomatic of ASD. Information regarding these questionnaires can be found in **Table 1**. Other questionnaires that are used to collect information regarding anxiety, behavior problems, overactivity, and other behaviors associated with conditions that can co-occur with ASD are included in the sections regarding co-occurring conditions.

Screeners, which are a subtype of questionnaires, serve the purpose of identifying individuals in the general population (level 1) or in at-risk populations (level 2) who should have additional testing to determine if ASD is present or not. Since early diagnosis can lead to early intervention, which can result in better outcomes for young children, guidelines for best practice for the process of screening for ASD were established in 2000 by a task group of ASD professionals.[47] After reviewing empirical evidence, the experts recommended that routine developmental surveillance and specific ASD screening be performed on all children, both to identify those at risk for any type of atypical development and to identify those specifically at risk for autism. Based on the results of the screening process, those at risk for ASD should be referred for a full diagnostic assessment. Despite the importance of early identification, almost 20 years have elapsed since the publication of these professional recommendations and guidelines and no population screening is yet in place in the United States. The American Academy of Pediatrics addressed this lack in its executive summary[48] providing 1 continuum for identification, evaluation, and management of ASD for primary care providers. This updated document begins with the importance of timely diagnosis, identification, and evidence-based intervention. The authors recommend using validated tools for general developmental screening as early as 9 months, continuing until 30 months. This ongoing developmental surveillance can help lower the age of diagnosis and facilitate earlier intervention.

Screening should be the first step leading to a more comprehensive diagnostic evaluation, but too often it is used in place of a complete evaluation and is related to as a diagnostic process rather than a beginning step. Specifically, screening measures used with the general population (level 1) must take into account both general developmental level as well as possible autism characteristics, whereas level 2 screening measures address specific autism symptomatology at very young ages. Level 2 screening measures have very low specificity and sensitivity, which means that they are identifying infants and toddlers with other developmental disabilities or issues as well as identifying the possibility of autism when the reported difficulties may stem from other developmental issues.[49] Screeners for ASD are presented in **Table 1**.

CO-OCCURRING CONDITIONS IN AUTISM SPECTRUM DISORDER

The co-occurrence of 2 or more clinical diagnoses, known as "comorbidity," has received much attention in the child psychopathology literature.[50] Because *DSM-5*[3] no longer excludes most additional diagnoses in children with ASD, an ASD diagnosis can coexist with many other conditions, a fact that has been recognized clinically. These additional problems have a substantial negative impact on functioning[51,52] and must be addressed as a crucial part of the diagnostic evaluation. Several large studies, most based on clinically referred samples, have reported that more than 70% of children with ASD were above diagnostic thresholds for another emotional or behavioral disorder and that more than 40% may have 2 or more comorbid mental health conditions,[53–56] including intellectual impairment.[57,58]

Co-occurring Conditions in Young Children

Most very young children who undergo an ASD assessment also have some general developmental delay. The complexity of understanding the overlap between ASD and ID is more pronounced in younger children, in whom distinguishing social communication limitations above and beyond the global developmental delays is difficult even for the most experienced clinicians.[59] Similarly, it is difficult to differentiate between ASD and developmental language disorder. The common features of individuals with ID and those with ID and ASD include cognitive and language delays, difficulties in behavioral regulation, aggressive outbursts, and/or self-injurious behavior. Although there are many similarities there are also some key distinctions that may be helpful in establishing a differential diagnosis. Often the cognitive profile of individuals with ID only will be more evenly distributed than the more scattered cognitive profile of individuals with ID and ASD. Likewise, although language and communication skills are delayed in ID without ASD, these young children experience fewer atypical behaviors and manifest more compensatory strategies. Social skills and adaptive functioning in individuals with ID tend to be similar to their mental age, whereas in individuals with ID and ASD they tend to be lower than expected based on mental age. Early history can also be quite informative for differential diagnosis. Parents of both groups often become concerned because of delayed language development or delayed crawling/walking,[59] but parents of children with ID and ASD also often describe social concerns, such as poor eye contact, limited social smiling, and difficulty engaging. Children with ID typically have appropriate eye contact and can play basic reciprocal games with adults. It is important when assessing cognitive abilities to remember that individuals with ASD have the most difficulty on tests involving the use of social and language skills, including attending to social information,[60–64] imitation,[65,66] and joint attention.[67] The scores on these types of tasks are likely to be lower than scores on tasks requiring skills that are often strengths in individuals with ASD (eg, perception, rote memory). This is particularly evident when testing very young children with ASD. For example, such children may have difficulty completing tasks that assess the ability to play reciprocal social games (eg, peek-a-boo), the ability to use an index finger to point to objects (eg, joint attention), and the ability to imitate the examiner's actions, which are the tasks frequently found in assessments designed to measure cognitive abilities in infants and toddlers. Thus, low scores on these cognitive measures may be associated with decreased attention, social engagement, and emotion regulation rather than true cognitive delays.[68] Although it may be impossible to find a test that does not involve these social and communication skills, an examiner should be aware of which tasks are likely to be particularly difficult for a child with ASD.

Co-occurring Conditions in School-Age Children, Adolescents, and Adults

Differential diagnosis in school-age children is complicated, as many of the conditions that commonly co-occur with ASD at this age also have substantial symptom overlap. Teasing out the student's interaction style from shyness to phobia to ASD can often be difficult without assessing all environments in which the student interacts with others. Generalized anxiety disorder (GAD), social phobia, obsessive-compulsive disorder, depression, and other mental health disorders need to be ruled out as a cause for the social deficits observed. This is where the diagnostic history interview becomes important, as it may help in understanding whether a youngster's current lack of social interaction is due to social anxiety, depression, or ASD.

Research has shown that throughout adolescence anxiety problems increase in students with ASD, especially in girls, whereas boys tend to have increased levels of depression,[69] which can exacerbate the social deficits associated with the ASD diagnosis. Depression has been reported to be a comorbid diagnosis in up to 65% of individuals with Asperger disorder,[70–76] along with higher levels of behavioral and emotional disturbances[77] and anxiety.[78,79] Attempts to commit suicide due to depressive symptoms are more frequent in individuals with higher functioning levels than is commonly recognized, especially when the individual reaches puberty and early adolescence.[80,81] Howlin[74] demonstrated that depression was the most common comorbid diagnosis provided to individuals with ASD during adulthood, yet these symptoms often began during adolescence. Peer victimization during early and mid-adolescence has been linked to higher rates of depression and anxiety[82] and has been correlated with higher rates of suicidal ideation,[83] and school-aged children with ASD are more likely to experience victimization than non-ASD children.[84–86] The relationship between bullying by peers and depressive symptoms has been well documented,[87] and it has been found in adolescents with ASD[88] as well as in those with typical development.

Although the cause of the impairments seen in students with ASD and GAD differs, many of the same skill deficits may be present in both disorders, such as difficulty communicating and interacting appropriately with others, poor eye contact and body posture, unusual speech quality, isolating behaviors, and difficulty building and maintaining friendships. Although people with ASD have issues with the basic elements of social communication and interactions that make relationships possible (eg, recognizing emotions and social cues in others), those with GAD may display social withdrawal due to excessive worry about the situation but their social cognition is intact. Someone with GAD may develop routines that seem rigid; however, it is often to gain a sense of control and/or avoid triggers. Gender and sexual identity issues may be an underlying factor in a school-age student's social skills deficits that may complicate the ASD assessment process. Social understanding is dependent on gender and sexuality identity, causing students to withdraw from social interactions with others when identity issues arise.

Like older children, adults with ASD have been found to have co-occurring psychiatric conditions at higher rates than the non-ASD population.[89] In contrast to typical development, males and females with ASD are reported to experience similar rates of co-occurring psychiatric conditions.[90] Thus, this is an area that must be addressed in any comprehensive evaluation of an individual with ASD. Dual diagnosis should be considered whenever there are signs of psychiatric problems that are not part of ASD; when there are marked changes in functioning from baseline or an existing problem is markedly exacerbated; or when an individual with ASD does not respond as expected to interventions that are have been found to be effective.[91] Assessment of co-occurring conditions is inherently complex and has presented a persistent challenge for both research and clinical work.[92]

Recognizing co-occurring conditions may also aid in the identification of underlying mechanisms, such as shared risk factors or 1 disorder creating a risk for another disorder. Developmental specialists involved in both clinical and research endeavors must be knowledgeable about the interplay between neurodevelopment and mental health issues, as the presentation of comorbid conditions results in more challenging assessments. Diagnosing ASD, with its broad range of symptom severity and intellectual functioning, is already a difficult task. Differences in clinical presentation that occur when there is more than 1 diagnostic entity add to the complexities of diagnostic assessment.

DIFFERENTIAL DIAGNOSIS AND CO-OCCURRING CONDITIONS

The behaviors that make up an ASD diagnosis may overlap with characteristics of other developmental and behavioral conditions and then the ability to differentiate among the disorders is particularly salient. It is imperative to address the differential diagnosis to understand whether an ASD diagnosis is appropriate or whether another condition better accounts for the profile revealed during the diagnostic evaluation. If another condition better accounts for the constellation of behaviors, then an ASD diagnosis is not warranted. However, it is possible for a person to manifest characteristics of ASD without meeting diagnostic threshold or for a person to meet diagnostic criteria for ASD and also have other diagnosable conditions. Characterizing and disentangling the symptom profiles by diagnostic criteria is a difficult but important process. The first step in understanding the overlap among symptoms is to obtain an extensive developmental history to examine the consistency of symptoms over time and their pervasiveness over contexts (for reviews see Mazefsky and colleagues[93,94]). If ASD is indeed the primary diagnosis, the core challenges in social communication and interaction should frame the person's interactions across situations and time, and the presence of restricted, repetitive, or unusual behaviors would support ASD as primary.

Attention-deficit/hyperactivity disorder (ADHD) presents an example of the necessity of extricating characteristics to establish whether ASD and ADHD co-occur in an individual or if one or the other diagnosis explains the presenting issues. Core features of ADHD include inattention, hyperactivity, and impulsivity,[3] and they may occur as part of ADHD or ASD or both in any given person. The coexistence of ASD and ADHD allows the clinician to respond to the fact that attention and hyperactivity are not always addressed by ASD interventions, whereas social understanding and decreasing repetitive and restrictive behaviors are not emphasized in ADHD interventions. Common features of ADHD and ASD include difficulties in listening to instructions, organization, and time management. ADHD in ASD may affect turn-taking and interrupting others (impulsivity), sitting still (hyperactivity), and understanding salient elements in the environment (attention). Most of these overlap with core impairments in ASD.[95] By examining the pervasiveness of symptoms across settings and the nature of the attentional problems, it may be possible to differentiate among them, but, with regard to anxiety, the clinician should be cautious in giving 2 diagnoses.[96] It has been suggested that the attentional problems in individuals with ADHD and those with ASD express themselves differently, with attention in ASD being more overfocused that in ADHD. It is necessary to conduct additional tests of attention that may provide clarity for differential diagnosis,[97] remembering that dual diagnoses can allow for effective treatments for the distinct impairments resulting from ADHD and ASD.

In addition, previous studies claimed that ASD and psychotic disorders may co-occur but that the rates are not more than would be expected to occur in the general population.[98] There is renewed interest in the overlap of schizophrenia and autism, but caution is required in interpreting this behavioral overlap because of a lack of empirical studies and some sample bias in studies based on psychiatric samples. To understand the co-occurrence of schizophrenia and ASD more information is needed, specifically empirical evidence that can be obtained through prospective developmental studies.

Finally, the impact of experiencing traumatic events on individuals with ASD is an area of increased clinical interest. Although the connection between trauma and anxiety and depression in neurotypical children and adults is well established,[99] scant research has been conducted regarding trauma in ASD.[100,101] Children with ASD may have increased vulnerability to trauma and victimization due to their increased dependence on adult caregivers, as well as their diagnosis-related difficulties with communication and social naiveté. Families of children with ASD may also experience increased stress that could increase the risk for maltreatment or traumatic events (eg, homelessness, placement outside the home).[100] Few studies have been conducted, but to date some evidence based on parent reports suggests an increased prevalence of adverse childhood experiences for children with ASD.[102,103] Research is only just emerging regarding signs and symptoms of trauma in children with ASD, and even less is available regarding evidence-based treatment.[101] A few studies have found that significant majorities (>80%) of adolescents and adults with ASD plus depression had experienced a traumatic event at some point in their lives.[104,105] These studies stress the importance of considering the contextual experiences of individuals with ASD and trauma during diagnosis and treatment.

Assessment of co-occurring conditions in ASD is inherently complicated and presents a persistent challenge for both researchers and clinicians.[106,107] Individuals may demonstrate mixed symptoms that stem from a single disorder with unusual presentation, or from the simultaneous occurrence of multiple disorders.[108] Although professionals are taught to think parsimoniously and make a single diagnosis whenever possible, it is important to note that an individual who meets diagnostic criteria for 1 mental health disorder is more likely to meet diagnostic criteria for another disorder than otherwise expected, supporting the claim that mental disorder constructs are correlated and dimensional.[109–111] Generally, those individuals who meet diagnostic criteria for more than 1 disorder manifest greater symptom severity and impairment than those who meet criteria for only 1 condition.[112,113] Developmental specialists involved in clinical work and research must be knowledgeable in both neurodevelopmental and mental health issues. The complexity of diagnosing ASD, with its heterogeneity in symptom severity, intellectual, language, and adaptive functioning, is already vast, and adding the need for differentiating dual diagnoses adds to the challenge. Although establishing differential diagnosis is a complex process, it is essential, because the coexistence of other problems may result in less than optimal responses to treatment.

As mentioned above, it is important to use standardized instruments in the diagnostic battery, but unfortunately, many behavior checklists and diagnostic interview tools were standardized in populations of children without ASD, making interpretation of scores challenging. It is not clear that norms developed for children without developmental disorders and with average cognitive functioning are relevant for children with ASD, with or without ID. Thus, it is sometimes hard to know whether children score in the clinical range on an instrument because they have ASD or because they are experiencing the particular difficulties that the tool measures. A second set of difficulties in assessing potential psychiatric problems in children with ASD with or without ID is limitations in the ability to process and talk about emotions and internal experiences.[114] In the assessment of psychopathology, the gold standard method is self-report, which can be problematic with individuals with ASD because of limitations in insight.[115] In addition, functional communication and pragmatic language skills may be limited. Response perseveration can also have an impact on self-report ratings.[116] For all these reasons, self-reporting of internal phenomena—essential to most assessments of psychopathology—may be less useful with children with ASD, especially those who are younger or lower functioning.[115] Thus, self-report measures should be used with caution when assessing individuals with ASD.

The most important complication in the assessment of co-occurring conditions in ASD is also the most challenging for the clinician and researcher. The range and quality of symptoms of other diagnostic categories can be influenced by the clinical expression of ASD. Symptoms of another condition may look different in the context of ASD, particularly in individuals with intellectual impairment.[50] It is possible that some people with ASD may not demonstrate certain symptoms, such as the feeling of guilt in depression, as a result of the social impairment at the core of ASD. Anxiety may manifest itself in someone with ASD as obsessive questioning or insistence on sameness rather than in rumination or somatic complaints.[117–119] Social responsiveness during an assessment is already impaired in ASD and therefore may be misinterpreted by professionals who are unfamiliar with ASD presentation, particularly in higher functioning, more capable individuals with ASD.

One way to address these issues and evaluate the presence of co-occurring conditions in ASD is to focus on changes in behavior from baseline. Significant changes in behavior from how the individual was described in the past—such as increases in social withdrawal, repetitive motor movements, aggression/outbursts, resistance to change, irritability, avoidance of novelty, or decreases in activities that once brought pleasure—can be crucial to making an accurate diagnosis,[91] although this can only be understood if one considers whether the frequency and the intensity of these behaviors are new or long-standing. Otherwise baseline exaggeration[120] may make the diagnostic distinctions less clear. For example, a newly noted decrease in the amount of time spent discussing a special interest (eg, the solar system, popular singers, or bus routes) may be helpful in recognizing the onset of a mood disorder in someone with a previous ASD diagnosis. In addition, the appearance of new challenging behaviors that have not been part of the clinical picture in the past, such as self-injury or aggression, will indicate the need for further evaluation. Unexplained decreases in self-care and other everyday living skills may also present diagnostic clues related to comorbidities in ASD. Comorbidity should be suspected when such changes from baseline are accompanied by significant clinical impairment in functioning and decreased adaptive behavior. Evaluations of risk factors (especially family history of comorbid conditions) and of environmental factors (eg, appropriate access to services and support) are other key elements in arriving at an accurate differential diagnosis.

Diagnostic formulation should involve questions regarding differential diagnosis: Does the individual have both ASD and another disorder, or just another disorder? For example, poor eye contact and low social initiative may be indicative of ASD, but also of depression. The first step in answering that question involves examination of the developmental history, looking for the consistency of symptoms over time. Social communication impairments appearing with odd, repetitive behaviors since childhood is indicative of ASD, as no other condition contains all those difficulties. If additional problems not encompassed by the ASD criteria are present, if there are changes from baseline indicating onset of new difficulties, or if the individual is not responding as expected to treatment, the possibility of a co-occurring condition should be considered.[91]

In summary, since there is increased risk of additional diagnoses of psychiatric disorders in people with ASD, including mood disorders, anxiety, depression, and schizophrenia,[121] instruments assessing psychiatric conditions should be included in an evaluation for ASD. This is particularly challenging as there is symptom overlap among ASD and psychiatric conditions. For example, 22% of adults with ASD also meet diagnostic criteria for anxiety disorder[122] and 25% of adults with ASD have clinical depression, whereas only 7% of the general population meet criteria for depression.[123] The difficulties in making a diagnostic decision arise not only from the overlapping symptomatology among psychiatric conditions and ASD (eg, dual diagnosis); there are also other nonspectrum conditions that present with impaired social functioning and thinking, such as schizophrenia, in which similar behavior profiles have been described (eg, differential diagnosis). In a research study examining the behavioral overlap between autism symptomatology in autism and schizophrenia, Maddox and colleagues[124] found that the ADOS-2 has a high false-positive rate for schizophrenia, despite that the revised algorithm module 4 (appropriate for adults with fluent language) now has 90.5% sensitivity and 82.2% specificity.[125] A complicated but understudied area of diagnostic complexity is the behavioral overlap with Personality and/or Thought disorders. Because these conditions typically are not evident until early adulthood, some unusual social and other behavior that manifested earlier in childhood as "odd" may become a profile of a Personality or Thought Disorder with or without ASD. The inclusion of professionals with training and experience in assessing psychiatric conditions is necessary when evaluating individuals for an ASD diagnosis in adulthood.

Several large research studies have shown that anxiety increases in age in individuals with ASD.[69] The reported rates in adults with ASD are well above those in the general population for all types of anxiety disorders (eg, GAD, social phobia and other phobias, and separation anxiety). It has been suggested that individuals with ASD are at greater risk for anxiety disorders because an expression of their ASD is incomprehension or miscomprehension of certain phenomena, which causes them to experience anxiety.[126] Irritability is often a manifestation of an anxiety disorder in ASD[127] and fewer social supports are available for adults with ASD. Although there is empirical evidence that anxiety symptoms are raised in individuals with ASD, it is important to recognize that there is clear overlap between the core behaviors of ASD and some anxiety disorders (eg, social phobia), which necessitates careful assessment as to whether an additional diagnosis is necessary. Mood disorders are the most commonly reported mental health problem in adults with ASD. This has been supported by the results from large population-based studies. Danish[128,129] and US[130] samples revealed co-occurring depression and ASD above rates in the general population. To differentiate symptoms associated with ASD and those associated with depression and to understand the symptom expression in individuals with ASD and with depression, Lainhart[91] identified new or worsening aggression, agitation, or an increase in obsessive-compulsive behaviors as the presenting complaint rather than something related to mood. It is important to note that individuals with ASD have difficulty expressing their emotional states and therefore depressed mood may not be the presenting symptom.[127] Increases in irritability and sleep disturbances may be alternative expressions of the sadness reported in individuals without ASD.

INSTRUMENTS FOR ASSESSING PSYCHIATRIC CO-OCCURRING CONDITIONS IN AUTISM SPECTRUM DISORDER

There are instruments that have been used in the ASD population to assess psychiatric status and these are presented below. It is clear from the list that there is a need to develop more specific instruments to understand the overlap of symptomatology among psychiatric and neurodevelopmental disorders, specifically ASD. Using these standardized instruments, we can begin to standardize diagnostic protocols and batteries when establishing dual diagnosis and differential diagnosis.

The Achenbach System of Empirically Based Assessment (ASEBA) evaluates behavior across the lifespan and includes forms for self-reporting and reporting from parents and teachers.[131] It measures symptoms of depression, anxiety, somatic complaints, obsessive-compulsive behaviors, attentional problems, social difficulties, aggression, and atypicalities in thinking. The version for young children also provides diagnostic criteria for ASD, and it has been shown effective in differentiating ASD from other psychiatric conditions[132,133] and has also been used to study co-occurring psychiatric conditions in ASD (see, for example, Almansour and colleagues,[134] Lohr and colleagues,[135] Lord and colleagues,[136] Stratis and Lecavalier,[137] Vaillancourt and colleagues,[138] and Visser and colleagues[139]). The community (ABC-Community[140]) is a 58-item behavior checklist completed by parents, teachers, or clinicians to evaluate problems encountered within the past month. Although it has been used to assess change as a result of intervention, specifically after pharmacologic research, some questions have arisen recently regarding its utility in assessing psychiatric conditions in individuals with ASD.[141–143] A useful tool for rapid screening for a variety of forms of psychopathology is the Child and Adolescent Symptom Inventory (CASI[144]). The fifth edition of this instrument has been updated with the *DSM-5* criteria and cutoffs are provided for all *DSM-5* conditions that appear in childhood and adolescence, and it has been used extensively to examine psychiatric comorbidities in ASD.[55,145–150]

The National Institute for Health and Care Excellence in the United Kingdom (https://www.nice.org.uk/guidance/cg142) has published recommendations for evaluations of ASD in adulthood, which include recommended instruments for adult assessment dependent on the individual's level of intellectual functioning. For those without ID the Autism-Spectrum Quotient and the Empathy Quotient, which are self-report measures, and the Asperger Syndrome Diagnostic Interview, are recommended. For individuals with ID, the recommendation is to use the ADOS-2 and the ADI-R, which are both included in the recommendations for those without ID also. The use of the ADI-R raises the issue that when seeing an adult there is often limited access to early developmental history or school records or even other third-party information regarding whether there have been developmental challenges, and if so what they were. Parents may not be available or in contact with the individual and it may be intrusive to try to gather developmental information from a third party.

SUMMARY AND FUTURE DIRECTIONS

There has been tremendous progress in understanding the importance of accurate diagnosis of ASD throughout the lifespan. Toward this goal, many tools have been developed for assessing ASD from early childhood through adulthood. The diagnosis and assessment of ASD is often challenging, even for experienced professionals, necessitating the integration of information from multiple sources, including a comprehensive developmental, medical, and behavioral history. Direct observation provides additional information without which the diagnosis cannot be made. Formal evaluations should depend on standardized instruments designed to measure social functioning, communication and language abilities, adaptive behavior, emotional functioning, and cognitive abilities. Only by gathering information across domains, including information about possible co-occurring conditions, may a comprehensive diagnostic profile be obtained. Comprehensive ASD assessment is important to provide an individually tailored intervention program for the person with ASD. Once an accurate diagnosis is obtained, understanding can begin to lead toward treatment and enhance the likelihood of positive outcomes for individuals with ASD and their families.

Although diagnosis can be established earlier than ever before, several issues remain underaddressed. The issues raised throughout this article deal with the need for knowledge and training in development and mental health in general, and in ASD specifically, which requires not simply training in the use of gold standard instruments but also in understanding ASD, as well as the overlap with other possible conditions, which may require dual diagnosis or differential diagnosis. Evaluation of co-occurring conditions in ASD challenges the best of clinicians and teasing out the core symptoms of ASD from other conditions is a complex undertaking. Clinicians must remember that apparent comorbidity may arise from overlapping behavioral symptoms and that one syndrome may represent an early manifestation of another disorder (eg, Rett syndrome). Better understanding of co-occurring conditions in ASD can help in understanding the heterogeneity and perhaps offer one possibility for meaningful subgrouping within ASD. Conditions that commonly co-occur may provide clues about shared risk factors or shared neurogenesis.

Perhaps the issue of measurement remains the most significant challenge for clinical diagnosticians and researchers alike. The existing instruments were not necessarily normed on individuals with ASD, and even when ASD norms exist there are limited normative data. One goal for future development is to be aware of the importance of deciding which comparison groups should be included in instrument development. It is essential to have standardized norms for individuals with typical development and other overlapping conditions, as well as groups of individuals with autism in the validation samples of instruments, to be able to differentiate among the different conditions. Similarly, the inadequacy of some of the existing instruments in terms of sensitivity and specificity results in missing some individuals with ASD and others receiving an ASD diagnosis when perhaps another diagnosis would lead to more effective intervention. Of late, both researchers and clinicians have focused more than previously on potential underdiagnosis of females, reinforcing the need for specification in existing diagnostic tools.[151] Increasing the sensitivity to the heterogeneity of ASD manifestation may be accomplished by using several instruments in the diagnostic battery, gathering information from various sources, and including evaluation of different functional domains by a multidisciplinary team of professionals.

Research and clinical practice converge in the need for accurate diagnosis and assessment in ASD. Current diagnostic and assessment tools allow for a reliable and valid diagnosis early in life and provide the foundation for studying developmental trajectories with different behavioral profiles and outcomes in an attempt to find meaningful subgroups of ASD, which could serve as a basis for streamlining interventions. Future research should include the study of diagnostic biomarkers for ASD and seek to establish more ecologically valid means of assessing the ways in which individuals with ASD function in adolescence and adulthood. In addition, the development of screeners which have better sensitivity and specificity would fill a void left by the existing instruments. There is still a need for characterization of underidentified and underdiagnosed groups including females, in whom some ASD symptomatology is expressed differently, and/or less severely, and higher functioning adults, who often are misdiagnosed with mental health problems only, overlooking the possibility of a dual diagnosis of ASD.

Having an accurate diagnosis can help people with ASD and their families because it can make sense of some of the differences they are seeing in behavior and development, as well as providing help by establishing appropriate expectations, learning from others who have experienced receiving a diagnosis of ASD for themselves or a family member. Information about the diagnosis can also protect people with ASD and their families from possible negative responses from others. The importance of an accurate diagnosis in providing information needed for accessing appropriate services and in facilitating communication among practitioners, professionals, researchers, and families cannot be overstated. Accurate diagnosis can also ensure comparability among participants assessed in different research studies and clinical settings to help understand developmental trajectories and the significance of changes over time, clarifying the similarities and differences which emerge during the life of any particular individual with ASD.

DISCLOSURE

The authors have nothing to disclose.

REFERENCES

1. Georgiades S, Bishop SL, Frazier T. Editorial Perspective: longitudinal research in autism–introducing the concept of 'chronogeneity'. J Child Psychol Psychiatry 2017;58(5):634–6.
2. Kanner L. Autistic disturbances of affective contact. Nervous Child 1943;2(3): 217–50.
3. American Psychiatric Association. Diagnostic and statistical manual of mental disorders. 5th edition. Washington, DC: American Psychiatric Association; 2013.
4. Mukaetova-Ladinska EB, Perry E, Baron M, et al, Autism Ageing Writing Group. Ageing in people with autistic spectrum disorder. Int J Geriatr Psychiatry 2012; 27(2):109–18.
5. Stuart-Hamilton I, Morgan H. What happens to people with autism spectrum disorders in middle age and beyond? Report of a preliminary on-line study. Adv Ment Health Intellect Disabil 2011;5(2):22–8.
6. Thomas KC, Ellis AR, McLaurin C, et al. Access to care for autism-related services. J Autism Dev Disord 2007;37(10):1902–12.
7. Ozonoff S, Goodlin-Jones BL, Solomon M. Evidence-based assessment of autism spectrum disorders in children and adolescents. J Clin Child Adolesc Psychol 2005;34(3):523–40.
8. Ozonoff S, Young GS, Brian J, et al. Diagnosis of autism spectrum disorder after age 5 in children evaluated longitudinally since infancy. J Am Acad Child Adolesc Psychiatry 2018;57(11):849–57.
9. Pedersen AL, Pettygrove S, Lu Z, et al. DSM criteria that best differentiate intellectual disability from autism spectrum disorder. Child Psychiatry Hum Dev 2017;48(4):537–45.
10. Robins DL, Fein D, Barton ML, et al. The Modified Checklist for Autism in Toddlers: an initial study investigating the early detection of autism and pervasive developmental disorders. J Autism Dev Disord 2001;31(2):131–44.
11. Snow AV, Lecavalier L. Sensitivity and specificity of the modified checklist for autism in toddlers and the social communication questionnaire in preschoolers

suspected of having pervasive developmental disorders. Autism 2008;12(6): 627–44.

12. Eaves LC, Wingert H, Ho HH. Screening for autism: agreement with diagnosis. Autism 2006;10(3):229–42.

13. Matson JL, Kozlowski AM, Fitzgerald ME, et al. True versus false positives and negatives on the modified checklist for autism in toddlers. Res Autism Spectr Disord 2013;7(1):17–22.

14. Sikora DM, Hall TA, Hartley SL, et al. Does parent report of behavior differ across ADOS-G classifications: analysis of scores from the CBCL and GARS. J Autism Dev Disord 2008;38(3):440–8.

15. Lecavalier. An evaluation of the Gilliam autism rating scale. J Autism Dev Disord 2005;35(6):795.

16. Berument SK, Rutter M, Lord C, et al. Autism screening questionnaire: diagnostic validity. Br J Psychiatry 1999;175(5):444–51.

17. Bishop SL, Hus V, Duncan A, et al. Subcategories of restricted and repetitive behaviors in children with autism spectrum disorders. J Autism Dev Disord 2013; 43(6):1287–97.

18. Chandler S, Charman T, Baird G, et al. Validation of the Social Communication Questionnaire in a population cohort of children with autism spectrum disorders. J Am Acad Child Adolesc Psychiatry 2007;46(10):1324–32.

19. Chandrasekhar T, Sikich L. Challenges in the diagnosis and treatment of depression in autism spectrum disorders across the lifespan. Dialogues Clin Neurosci 2015;17(2):219.

20. Charman T, Taylor E, Drew A, et al. Outcome at 7 years of children diagnosed with autism at age 2: predictive validity of assessments conducted at 2 and 3 years of age and pattern of symptom change over time. J Child Psychol Psychiatry 2005;46(5):500–13.

21. Chlebowski C, Green JA, Barton ML, et al. Using the childhood autism rating scale to diagnose autism spectrum disorders. J Autism Dev Disord 2010; 40(7):787–99.

22. Clark MLE, Vinen Z, Barbaro J, et al. School age outcomes of children diagnosed early and later with autism spectrum disorder. J Autism Dev Disord 2018;48(1):92–102.

23. Corsello C, Hus V, Pickles A, et al. Between a ROC and a hard place: decision making and making decisions about using the SCQ. J Child Psychol Psychiatry 2007;48(9):932–40.

24. Witwer AN, Lecavalier L. Autism screening tools: an evaluation of the social communication questionnaire and the developmental behaviour checklist–autism screening algorithm. J Intellect Dev Disabil 2007;32(3):179–87.

25. Witwer AN, Lecavalier L. Validity of comorbid psychiatric disorders in youngsters with autism spectrum disorders. J Dev Phys Disabil 2010;22(4):367–80.

26. Zablotsky B, Bradshaw CP, Anderson CM, et al. Risk factors for bullying among children with autism spectrum disorders. Autism 2014;18:419–27.

27. Zander E, Sturm H, Bölte S. The added value of the combined use of the Autism Diagnostic Interview–Revised and the Autism Diagnostic Observation Schedule: diagnostic validity in a clinical Swedish sample of toddlers and young preschoolers. Autism 2015;19(2):187–99.

28. Constantino JN, Lavesser PD, Zhang YI, et al. Rapid quantitative assessment of autistic social impairment by classroom teachers. J Am Acad Child Adolesc Psychiatry 2007;46(12):1668–76.

29. Aldridge FJ, Gibbs VM, Schmidhofer K, et al. Investigating the clinical useful-ness of the Social Responsiveness Scale (SRS) in a tertiary level, autism spec-trum disorder specific assessment clinic. J Autism Dev Disord 2012;42(2): 294–300.

30. Cholemkery H, Kitzerow J, Rohrmann S, et al. Validity of the Social Responsive-ness Scale to differentiate between autism spectrum disorders and disruptive behaviour disorders. Eur Child Adolesc Psychiatry 2014;23(2):81–93.

31. Goldstein S, Naglieri JA. Autism spectrum rating scales (ASRS) technical manual. New York: Multi-Health Systems; 2013.

32. Goldstein S, Ozonoff S, editors. Assessment of autism spectrum disorder. New York: Guilford Publications; 2018.

33. Gotham K, Risi S, Pickles A, et al. The Autism Diagnostic Observation Schedule: revised algorithms for improved diagnostic validity. J Autism Dev Disord 2007; 37(4):613.

34. Gotham K, Risi S, Dawson G, et al. A replication of the autism diagnostic obser-vation schedule (ADOS) revised algorithms. J Am Acad Child Adolesc Psychi-atry 2008;47(6):642–51.

35. Zhou H, Zhang L, Luo X, et al. Modifying the autism spectrum rating scale (6–18 years) to a Chinese context: an exploratory factor analysis. Neurosci Bull 2017; 33(2):175–82.

36. Zwaigenbaum L, Bauman ML, Stone WL, et al. Early identification of autism spectrum disorder: recommendations for practice and research. Pediatrics 2015;136(Supplement 1):S10–40.

37. Camodeca A. Description of criterion validity of the autism spectrum rating scales 6–18 parent report: initial exploration in a large community sample. Child Psychiatry Hum Dev 2019;50(6):987–1001.

38. Lord C, Luyster R, Guthrie W, et al. Patterns of developmental trajectories in tod-dlers with autism spectrum disorder. J Consult Clin Psychol 2012;80(3):477.

39. Lord C, Corsello C, Grzadzinski R. Diagnostic instruments in autism spectrum disorders. In: Volkmar FR, Rogers S, Paul R, et al, editors. Handbook of autism and pervasive developmental disorders. 4th edition. New Jersey: John Wiley and Sons; 2014. p. 609–60.

40. Luyster R, Gotham K, Guthrie W, et al. The Autism Diagnostic Observation Schedule—Toddler Module: a new module of a standardized diagnostic mea-sure for autism spectrum disorders. J Autism Dev Disord 2009;39(9):1305–20.

41. Pfeffer RD. Childhood victimization in a national sample of youth with autism spectrum disorders. J Policy Pract Intellect Disabil 2016;13(4):311–9.

42. Rapin I, Dunn M. Update on the language disorders of individuals on the autistic spectrum. Brain Dev 2003;25(3):166–72.

43. Richler J, Bishop SL, Kleinke JR, et al. Restricted and repetitive behaviors in young children with autism spectrum disorders. J Autism Dev Disord 2007; 37(1):73–85.

44. Risi S, Lord C, Gotham K, et al. Combining information from multiple sources in the diagnosis of autism spectrum disorders. J Am Acad Child Adolesc Psychi-atry 2006;45(9):1094–103.

45. Rutter M, Le Couteur A, Lord C. Autism diagnostic interview-revised. Los An-geles (CA): Western Psychological Services; 2003. p. 29, 30.

46. Schopler E, Reichler RJ, Renner BR. The childhood autism rating scale (CARS). Los Angeles (CA): WPS; 2010.

47. Filipek PA, Accardo PJ, Ashwal S, et al. Practice parameter: screening and diagnosis of autism: report of the quality standards subcommittee of the

American Academy of Neurology and the Child Neurology Society. Neurology 2000;55(4):468–79.

48. Hyman SL, Levy SE, Myers SM. Identification, evaluation, and management of children with autism spectrum disorder. Pediatrics 2019. https://doi.org/10.1542/peds.2019-3447.

49. Norris M, Lecavalier L. Screening accuracy of level 2 autism spectrum disorder rating scales: a review of selected instruments. Autism 2010;14(4):263–84.

50. Cervantes PE, Matson JL. Comorbid symptomology in adults with autism spectrum disorder and intellectual disability. J Autism Dev Disord 2015;45(12): 3961–70.

51. Lecavalier L. An evaluation of the Gilliam autism rating scale. J Autism Dev Disord 2006;35(6):795.

52. Lee HJ. Cultural factors related to the hidden curriculum for students with autism and related disabilities. Interv Sch Clin 2011;46(3):141–9.

53. Gjevik E, Eldevik S, Fjæran-Granum T, et al. Kiddie-SADS reveals high rates of DSM-IV disorders in children and adolescents with autism spectrum disorders. J Autism Dev Disord 2011;41(6):761–9.

54. Joshi G, Wozniak J, Petty C, et al. Psychiatric comorbidity and functioning in a clinically referred population of adults with autism spectrum disorders: a comparative study. J Autism Dev Disord 2013;43(6):1314–25.

55. Kaat AJ, Gadow KD, Lecavalier L. Psychiatric symptom impairment in children with autism spectrum disorders. J Abnorm Child Psychol 2013;41(6):959–69.

56. Simonoff E, Pickles A, Charman T, et al. Psychiatric disorders in children with autism spectrum disorders: prevalence, co-morbidity, and associated factors in a population-derived sample. J Am Acad Child Adolesc Psychiatry 2008; 47(8):921–9.

57. Rydzewska E, Hughes-McCormack LA, Gillberg C, et al. Prevalence of sensory impairments, physical and intellectual disabilities, and mental health in children and young people with self/proxy-reported autism: observational study of a whole country population. Autism 2019;23(5):1201–9.

58. Schopler E, Richter RJ, DeVellis RF, et al. Toward objective classification of childhood autism: Childhood Autism Rating Scale (CARS). J Autism Dev Disord 1980;10:91–103.

59. Bishop SL, Thurm A, Farmer C, et al. Autism spectrum disorder, intellectual disability, and delayed walking. Pediatrics 2016;137(3):e20152959.

60. Dawson G, Toth K, Abbott R, et al. Early social attention impairments in autism: social orienting, joint attention, and attention to distress. Dev Psychol 2004; 40(2):271.

61. Dawson G. Early behavioral intervention, brain plasticity, and the prevention of autism spectrum disorder. Dev Psychopathol 2008;20(03):775–803.

62. Dawson G, Rogers SJ, Munson J, et al. Randomized, controlled trial of an intervention for toddlers with autism: the early start Denver model. Pediatrics 2010; 125:17–23.

63. Dawson G, Jones EJ, Merkle K, et al. Early behavioral intervention is associated with normalized brain activity in young children with autism. J Am Acad Child Adolesc Psychiatry 2012;51:1150–9.

64. de Bildt A, Sytema S, van Lang ND, et al. Evaluation of the ADOS revised algorithm: the applicability in 558 Dutch children and adolescents. J Autism Dev Disord 2009;39(9):1350–8.

65. Rogers SJ, Hepburn SL, Stackhouse T, et al. Imitation performance in toddlers with autism and those with other developmental disorders. J Child Psychol Psychiatry 2003;44(5):763–81.
66. Rutter M. The development of infantile autism. Psychol Med 1974;4:147–63.
67. Mundy P, Sigman M, Kasari C. Joint attention, developmental level, and symptom presentation in autism. Dev Psychopathol 1994;6(3):389–401.
68. Burns CO, Matson JL, Cervantes PE, et al. Hearing impairment, autism spectrum disorder, and developmental functioning in infants and toddlers. J Dev Phys Disabil 2016;28(4):495–507.
69. Gotham K, Brunwasser SM, Lord C. Depressive and anxiety symptom trajectories from school age through young adulthood in samples with autism spectrum disorder and developmental delay. J Am Acad Child Adolesc Psychiatry 2015;54(5):369–76.
70. Ellis HD, Ellis DM, Fraser W, et al. A preliminary study of right hemisphere cognitive deficits and impaired social judgments among young people with Asperger syndrome. Eur Child Adolesc Psychiatry 1994;3:255–66.
71. Ghaziuddin M, Ghaziuddin N, Greden J. Depression in persons with autism: implications for research and clinical care. J Autism Dev Disord 2002;32:299–306.
72. Green J, Gilchrist A, Burton D, et al. Social and psychiatric functioning in adolescents with Asperger syndrome compared with conduct disorder. J Autism Dev Disord 2000;30:279–93.
73. Grzadzinski R, Huerta M, Lord C. DSM-5 and autism spectrum disorders (ASDs): an opportunity for identifying ASD subtypes. Mol Autism 2013; 4(1):12–7.
74. Howlin P. Outcomes in autism spectrum disorders. In: Volkmar FR, Paul R, Klin A, et al, editors. Handbook of autism and pervasive developmental disorders. Diagnosis, development, neurobiology, and behavior, vol. 1, 3rd edition. Hoboken (NJ): John Wiley & Sons; 2005. p. 201–20.
75. Howlin P, Moss P, Savage S, et al. Social outcomes in mid-to later adulthood among individuals diagnosed with autism and average nonverbal IQ as children. J Am Acad Child Adolesc Psychiatry 2013;52(6):572–81.
76. Huerta M, Lord C. Diagnostic evaluation of autism spectrum disorders. Pediatr Clin North Am 2012;59(1):103–11.
77. Tonge BJ, Brereton AV, Gray KM, et al. Behavioural and emotional disturbance in high-functioning autism and Asperger syndrome. Autism 1999;3:117–30.
78. White SW, Roberson-Nay R. Anxiety, social deficits, and loneliness in youth with autism spectrum disorders. J Autism Dev Disord 2009;39:1006–13.
79. White SW, Oswald D, Ollendick T, et al. Anxiety in children and adolescents with autism spectrum disorders. Clin Psychol Rev 2009;29:216–29.
80. Fitzgerald M. Editorial: suicide and Asperger's syndrome. Crisis 2007;28:1–3.
81. Gillberg C. A guide to Asperger's syndrome. Cambridge (England): Cambridge University Press; 2002.
82. Stapinski LA, Araya R, Heron J, et al. Peer victimization during adolescence: concurrent and prospective impact on symptoms of depression and anxiety. Anxiety Stress Coping 2015;28(1):105–20.
83. Cleary SD. Adolescent victimization and associated suicidal and violent behaviors. Adolescence 2000;35:671–82.
84. Forrest DL, Kroeger RA, Stroope S. Autism spectrum disorder symptoms and bullying victimization among children with autism in the United States. J Autism Dev Disord 2019;1–12. https://doi.org/10.1007/s10803-019-04282-9.

85. Framingham J. Minnesota multiphasic personality inventory (MMPI). Newbury Port (MA): Psych Central; 2018. Available at: https://psychcentral.com/lib/minnesota-multiphasic-personality-inventory-mmpi/. Accessed October 1, 2019.

86. Fusar-Poli L, Brondino N, Rocchetti M, et al. Diagnosing ASD in adults without ID: accuracy of the ADOS-2 and the ADI-R. J Autism Dev Disord 2017;47(11):3370–9.

87. Seals D, Young J. Bullying and victimization: prevalence and relationship to gender, grade level, ethnicity, self-esteem, and depression. Adolescence 2003;38(152):735–47.

88. Shtayermman O. Peer victimization in adolescents and young adults diagnosed with Asperger's syndrome: a link to depressive symptomatology, anxiety symptomatology, and suicidal ideation. Issues Compr Pediatr Nurs 2007;30:87–107.

89. Deprey L, Ozonoff S. Assessment of comorbid psychiatric conditions in autism spectrum disorder. In: S. Goldstein, S. Ozonoff, editors. Assessment of autism spectrum disorder. New York: Guilford Publications. 2018, 308-36.

90. Holtmann M, Bölte S, Poustka F. Autism spectrum disorders: sex differences in autistic behaviour domains and coexisting psychopathology. Dev Med Child Neurol 2007;49(5):361–6.

91. Lainhart JE. Psychiatric problems in individuals with autism, their parents and siblings. Int Rev Psychiatry 1999;11(4):278–98.

92. Krueger RF, Markon KE. Reinterpreting comorbidity: a model-based approach to understanding and classifying psychopathology. Annu Rev Clin Psychol 2006;27:111–33.

93. Mazefsky CA, Pelphrey KA, Dahl RE. The need for a broader approach to emotion regulation research in autism. Child Dev Perspect 2012;6(1):92–7.

94. Mazefsky CA, Herrington J, Siegel M, et al. The role of emotion regulation in autism spectrum disorder. J Am Acad Child Adolesc Psychiatry 2013;52(7):679–88.

95. Grzadzinski R, Dick C, Lord C, et al. Parent-reported and clinician-observed autism spectrum disorder (ASD) symptoms in children with attention deficit/hyperactivity disorder (ADHD): implications for practice under DSM-5. Mol Autism 2016;7(1):7.

96. Muskens JB, Velders FP, Staal WG. Medical comorbidities in children and adolescents with autism spectrum disorders and attention deficit hyperactivity disorders: a systematic review. European Child & Adolescent Psychiatry 2017;26(9):1093–103.

97. Sutoko S, Monden Y, Tokuda T, et al. Distinct methylphenidate-evoked response measured using functional near-infrared spectroscopy during Go/No-Go task as a supporting differential diagnostic tool between Attention-Deficit/Hyperactivity Disorder and Autism Spectrum Disorder comorbid children. Front Hum Neurosci 2019;13:7.

98. Kincaid DL, Doris M, Shannon C, et al. What is the prevalence of autism spectrum disorder and ASD traits in psychosis? A systematic review. Psychiatry Res 2017;250:99–105.

99. Copeland WE, Keelar G, Angold A, et al. Traumatic events and posttraumatic stress in childhood. Arch Gen Psychiatry 2007;64:577–84.

100. Kerns C, Newschaffer C, Berkowitz S. Traumatic childhood events and autism spectrum disorder. J Autism Dev Disord 2015;45(11):3475–86.

101. Stack A, Lucyshyn J. Autism spectrum disorder and the experience of traumatic events: review of the current literature to inform modifications to a treatment model for children with autism. J Autism Dev Disord 2019;49(4):1613–25.
102. Berg KL, Shiu CS, Acharya K, et al. Disparities in adversity among children with autism spectrum disorder: a population-based study. Dev Med Child Neurol 2016;58:1124–31.
103. Kerns C, Newschaffer C, Berkowitz S, et al. Brief report: examining the association of autism and adverse childhood experiences in the national survey of children's health: the important role of income and co-occurring mental health conditions. J Autism Dev Disord 2017;47:2275–81.
104. Ghaziuddin M, Alessi N, Greden JF. Life events and depression in children with pervasive developmental disorders. J Autism Dev Disord 1995;25(5):495–502.
105. Taylor JL, Gotham KO. Cumulative life events, traumatic experiences, and psychiatric symptomatology in transition-aged youth with autism spectrum disorder. J Neurodev Disord 2016;8(1):28.
106. Bertelli MO, Underwood L, McCarthy J, et al. Assessment and diagnosis of psychiatric disorder in adults with autism spectrum disorder. Adv Ment Health Intellect Disabil 2015;9:222–9.
107. Moss P, Howlin P, Savage S, et al. Self and informant reports of mental health difficulties among adults with autism findings from a long-term follow-up study. Autism 2015;19(7):832–41.
108. Lyall K, Croen L, Daniels J, et al. The changing epidemiology of autism spectrum disorders. Annu Rev Public Health 2017;38:81–102.
109. Constantino JN. The quantitative nature of autistic social impairment. Pediatr Res 2011;69(5 Pt 2):55R–62R.
110. Constantino JN, Gruber CP. Social responsiveness scale–second edition (SRS-2). Torrance (CA): Western Psychological Services; 2012.
111. Constantino JN, Charman T. Diagnosis of autism spectrum disorder: reconciling the syndrome, its diverse origins, and variation in expression. Lancet Neurol 2016;15(3):279–91.
112. Rutter M. Changing concepts and findings on autism. J Autism Dev Disord 2013;43(8):1749–57.
113. Gadow KD, Guttmann-Steinmetz S, Rieffe C, et al. Depression symptoms in boys with autism spectrum disorder and comparison samples. J Autism Dev Disord 2012;42(7):1353–63.
114. Eack SM, Mazefsky CA, Minshew NJ. Misinterpretation of facial expressions of emotion in verbal adults with autism spectrum disorder. Autism 2015;19(3):308–15.
115. Mazefsky CA, Kao J, Oswald DP. Preliminary evidence suggesting caution in the use of psychiatric self-report measures with adolescents with high-functioning autism spectrum disorder. Res Autism Spectr Disord 2011;5(1):164–74.
116. Ben Shalom DB, Mostofsky SH, Hazlett RL, et al. Normal physiological emotions but differences in expression of conscious feelings in children with high-functioning autism. J Autism Dev Disord 2006;36(3):395–400.
117. Kerns CM, Rump K, Worley J, et al. The differential diagnosis of anxiety disorders in cognitively-able youth with autism. Cogn Behav Pract 2016;23(4):530–47.
118. Kiely KM, Butterworth P. Validation of four measures of mental health against depression and generalized anxiety in a community based sample. Psychiatry Res 2015;225(3):291–8.

119. Kim SH, Thurm A, Shumway S, et al. Multisite study of new autism diagnostic interview-revised (ADI-R) algorithms for toddlers and young preschoolers. J autism Dev Disord 2013;43(7):1527–38.

120. Ferrell RB, Wolinsky EJ, Kauffman CI, et al. Neuropsychiatric syndromes in adults with intellectual disability: issues in assessment and treatment. Curr Psychiatry Rep 2004;6(5):380–90.

121. Croen LA, Zerbo O, Qian Y, et al. The health status of adults on the autism spectrum. Autism 2015;19(7):814–23.

122. Gillberg IC, Helles A, Billstedt E, et al. Boys with Asperger syndrome grow up: psychiatric and neurodevelopmental disorders 20 years after initial diagnosis. J Autism Dev Disord 2016;46(1):74–82.

123. Matheis M, Turygin NC. Depression and autism. In: Matson J, editor. Handbook of assessment and diagnosis of autism spectrum disorder. New York: Springer; 2016. p. 285–300.

124. Maddox BB, Brodkin ES, Calkins ME, et al. The accuracy of the ADOS-2 in identifying autism among adults with complex psychiatric conditions. J Autism Dev Disord 2017;47(9):2703–9.

125. Hus V, Lord C. The autism diagnostic observation schedule, module 4: revised algorithm and standardized severity scores. J Autism Dev Disord 2014;44(8): 1996–2012.

126. Burrows CA, Usher LV, Becker-Haimes EM, et al. Profiles and correlates of parent–child agreement on social anxiety symptoms in youth with autism spectrum disorder. J Autism Dev Disord 2018;48(6):2023–37.

127. Mayes SD, Calhoun SL, Murray MJ, et al. Anxiety, depression, and irritability in children with autism relative to other neuropsychiatric disorders and typical development. Res Autism Spectr Disord 2011;5(1):474–85.

128. Abdallah MW, Greaves-Lord K, Grove J, et al. Psychiatric comorbidities in autism spectrum disorders: findings from a Danish Historic Birth Cohort. Eur Child Adolesc Psychiatry 2011;20:599–601.

129. Achenbach TM, Rescorla LA, Maruish ME. The Achenbach system of empirically based assessment (ASEBA) for ages 1.5 to 18 years. In: Maruish ME, editor. The Use of Psychological Testing for Treatment Planning and Outcomes Assessment2. New York: Routledge; 2004. p. 179–213.

130. Close HA, Lee LC, Kaufmann CN, et al. Co-occurring conditions and change in diagnosis in autism spectrum disorders. Pediatrics 2012;129(2):e305–16.

131. Achenbach TM. The Achenbach system of empirically based assessment (ASEBA): development, findings, theory, and applications. Burlington (VT): University of Vermont, Research Center for Children, Youth, & Families; 2009.

132. Duarte CS, Bordin IA, De Oliveira A, et al. The CBCL and the identification of children with autism and related conditions in Brazil: pilot findings. J Autism Dev Disord 2003;33(6):703–7.

133. Petersen DJ, Bilenberg N, Hoerder K, et al. The population prevalence of child psychiatric disorders in Danish 8- to 9-year-old children. Eur Child Adolesc Psychiatry 2006;15(2):71–8.

134. Almansour MA, Alateeq MA, Alzahrani MK, et al. Depression and anxiety among parents and caregivers of autistic spectral disorder children. Neurosciences (Riyadh) 2013;18(1):58–63.

135. Lohr WD, Daniels K, Wiemken T, et al. The screen for child anxiety-related emotional disorders is sensitive but not specific in identifying anxiety in children with high-functioning autism spectrum disorder: a pilot comparison to the

Achenbach system of empirically based assessment scales. Front Psychiatry 2017;8:138.

136. Lord C, Risi S, DiLavore PS, et al. Autism from 2 to 9 years of age. Arch Gen Psychiatry 2006;63(6):694–701.

137. Stratis EA, Lecavalier L. Restricted and repetitive behaviors and psychiatric symptoms in youth with autism spectrum disorders. Res Autism Spectr Disord 2013;7(6):757–66.

138. Vaillancourt T, Haltigan JD, Smith I, et al. Joint trajectories of internalizing and externalizing problems in preschool children with autism spectrum disorder. Dev Psychopathol 2017;29(1):203–14.

139. Visser JC, Rommelse NN, Lappenschaar M, et al. Variation in the early trajectories of autism symptoms is related to the development of language, cognition, and behavior problems. J Am Acad Child Adolesc Psychiatry 2017;56(8): 659–68.

140. Aman MG, Singh N. Aberrant behavior checklist. Community (ABC). East Aurora (NY): Slosson Educational Publications; 1994.

141. Swineford L. Validity of the Aberrant Behavior Checklist. Poster presented at the INSAR conference in Montreal, CA, May 1-4, 2019.

142. Tachimori H, Osada H, Kurita H. Childhood autism rating Scale-Tokyo version for screening pervasive developmental disorders. Psychiatry Clin Neurosci 2003; 57(1):113–8.

143. Taylor LJ, Maybery MT, Grayndler L, et al. Evidence for shared deficits in identifying emotions from faces and from voices in autism spectrum disorders and specific language impairment. Int J Lang Commun Disord 2015;50(4):452–66.

144. Gadow K, Sprafkin J. Child and adolescent symptom inventory 4R: screening and norms manual. Stony Brook (NY): Checkmate Plus; 2010.

145. Bitsika V, Sharpley CF. The association between autism spectrum disorder symptoms in high-functioning male adolescents and their mothers' anxiety and depression. J Dev Phys Disabil 2017;29(3):461–73.

146. Brereton AV, Tonge BJ, Einfeld SL. Psychopathology in children and adolescents with autism compared to young people with intellectual disability. J Autism Dev Disord 2006;36(7):863–70.

147. Brett D, Warnell F, McConachie H, et al. Factors affecting age at ASD diagnosis in UK: no evidence that diagnosis age has decreased between 2004 and 2014. J Autism Dev Disord 2016;46(6):1974–84.

148. Bryson SE, Zwaigenbaum L, McDermott C, et al. The Autism Observation Scale for Infants: scale development and reliability data. J Autism Dev Disord 2008; 38(4):731–8.

149. Wolfers T, Floris DL, Dinga R, et al. From pattern classification to stratification: towards conceptualizing the heterogeneity of Autism Spectrum Disorder. Neuroscience & Biobehavioral Reviews 2019.

150. Leyfer OT, Folstein SE, Bacalman S, et al. Comorbid psychiatric disorders in children with autism: interview development and rates of disorders. J Autism Dev Disord 2006;36(7):849–61.

151. Lehnhardt FG, Falter CM, Gawronski A, et al. Sex-related cognitive profile in autism spectrum disorders diagnosed late in life: implications for the female autistic phenotype. J Autism Dev Disord 2016;46(1):139–54.

Current Approaches to the Pharmacologic Treatment of Core Symptoms Across the Lifespan of Autism Spectrum Disorder

Gahan Pandina, PhD[a],*, Robert H. Ring, PhD[b,1],
Abigail Bangerter, DEdPsy[a], Seth Ness, MD, PhD[a]

KEYWORDS

- ASD • Autism • Drug development • Therapeutics • Clinical trials

KEY POINTS

- The core symptoms of ASD have a devastating impact on functioning and quality of life across the lifespan. There are no approved medications for ASD core symptoms.
- Recent developments in the understanding of biologic basis of ASD have led to novel targets with the potential to impact core symptoms.
- Heterogeneity in course of development, co-occurring conditions, and age-related treatment response variability hampers study outcomes.
- Novel measures and approaches to ASD clinical trial design will be helpful in the development of effective pharmacologic treatments.

BACKGROUND

Autism is a lifelong neurodevelopmental disorder characterized by deficits in core areas of social communication and restricted and repetitive behaviors and interests. There are currently no approved medications for the core symptoms of autism spectrum disorder (ASD), although recent developments in the understanding of biologic models of ASD have led to identification of potential psychopharmacologic targets. Several factors hamper the advance of pharmacologic interventions for ASD. For example, heterogeneity in origin and presentation of symptoms can impact outcomes. In addition, symptom patterns can fluctuate over the course of development, with new

[a] Janssen Research & Development, LLC, 1125 Trenton Harbouron Road, Titusville, NJ 08560, USA; [b] Kaerus Bioscience Ltd, London, UK
[1] Present address: 2110 South Eagle Road, Suite 392, Newtown, PA, 18940.
* Corresponding author.
E-mail address: gpandina@its.jnj.com

Child Adolesc Psychiatric Clin N Am 29 (2020) 301–317
https://doi.org/10.1016/j.chc.2019.12.004
1056-4993/20/© 2020 Elsevier Inc. All rights reserved.

childpsych.theclinics.com

ASD symptoms emerging across the lifespan, which must be accounted for to develop tools for and assess efficacy of psychopharmacologic interventions.

There is limited knowledge about the distribution and course of ASD symptoms across the lifespan.[1,2] Features of autism change over the course of development, with core symptom severity generally reported to reduce over time.[3–7] Recent studies have found that across the span of adulthood, main traits remain stable.[2] A 40-year longitudinal study has shown a general improvement in symptoms into young adulthood, but poorer outcomes in later adulthood.[8] Although core domains, on the whole, may reduce in severity across the lifespan, some symptom subdomains, such as restricted interests[7] or facial expression,[1] may be more stable over time. The impact of these long-term deficits on functioning is severe, with manifestations becoming increasingly complex later in life.[9] Large individual differences in trajectory are mediated by other factors, such as joint attention and language skills[1,10] and intellectual functioning.[7,11,12] In addition, environmental factors and the access to or availability of interventions influence the course of ASD.[13] Behavioral interventions have been shown to improve the core symptoms of ASD and change the trajectory of impact of ASD on functional outcome, particularly if started early.[14] In addition, there is evidence that behavioral interventions used in conjunction with careful medication management may be most effective.[15] Only two medications have been approved for associated symptoms (irritability) in ASD. Despite this, a systematic review indicated widespread use of prescription medication in ASD with a median prevalence of 41.9% in children and 61.5% in adults, with older age and psychiatric comorbidities associated with increased prescription medication use.[16] Atypical antipsychotics are most frequently used, followed by stimulant and nonstimulant attention-deficit/hyperactivity disorder medication and then antidepressants. However, there is variability in level of evidence available for the safety, tolerability, and effectiveness of many of these medications in ASD, particularly in adult populations.[17]

As evidence for the pathophysiology and neurobiology underlying core symptoms of ASD continues to grow, there is increasing interest in novel compounds that could impact crucial brain functions in autism, reducing symptoms, improving functioning, and potentially having an impact on long-term outcome. A review of active trials listed in the clinical trial registry, clinicaltrials.gov (as of November 2019), identified 51 current trials with the primary outcome listed as the core symptoms of ASD. Key targets cover a range of neurobiologic pathways: these range from glutamate and γ-aminobutyric acid (GABA), to neuroinflammation, immune responses, neuropeptides, and the endocannabinoid system (**Table 1**). Many of these clinical trials include children and/or younger adults, with fewer than 20% targeting symptoms in adults older than 30 years of age.

NEUROBIOLOGY AND PATHWAYS OF INTEREST FOR CORE SYMPTOMS
Glutamate and γ-Aminobutyric Acid

Perhaps the predominant and longest-standing theory of the neurobiology of ASD is the excitation-inhibition hypothesis, postulating an imbalance between glutamate and GABA.[18] Glutamate is an amino acid that functions as an excitatory neurotransmitter at a large proportion of synapses throughout the central nervous system (CNS) and is comprised of fast transmission ionotropic receptors (AMPA, N-methyl-D-aspartate [NMDA], and kainate), and slower, modulatory metabotropic receptors (three classes, I to IX). GABA is also an amino acid that functions as an inhibitory neurotransmitter. Although it seems that this theory should be highly explanatory, conflicting findings in the directionality of glutamate and GABA in humans and in animal

Table 1
Current targets in clinical trials for ASD

Trial Number	Target	Title	Age Range
Glutamate and GABA (including channelopathies)			
NCT02278328[a]	GABA-B	MEG Study of STX209	18–30 y
NCT03589898[a]	α2δ (VGCC)	Study of Neuroimaging Biomarkers of Social Cognition Deficits in Adolescents (Age 13–17) With ASD and Effects of Gabapentin	18–30 y
NCT03594552	GABA-B	Modulation of the Brain Excitatory/Inhibitory (E/I) Balance in Autism Spectrum Disorder (ASD)	**18–65 y**
NCT03678129	GABA-A	GABA Pathways in Autism Spectrum Disorder (ASD)	11–17 y
NCT03434366[b]	NR2A/NR2B	Intranasal Ketamine With Dexmedetomidine for the Treatment of Children With Autism Spectrum Disorder	2–4 y
NCT03682978[b]	GABA-B	Arbaclofen in Children and Adolescents With ASD	3–25 y
NCT03887676[b]	GABA-B	Arbaclofen vs Placebo in the Treatment of Children and Adolescents With ASD (ARBA)	3–7 y
NCT01813318[c]	GABA-A/NMDA-Rs	Study of Acamprosate in Autism	2–15 y
Inflammation and immunology			
NCT03826940	HMGCR	From Molecules to Cognition: Inhibitory Mechanisms in ASD and NF1	4–18 y
NCT02561481[b]	Antioxidant	Sulforaphane Treatment of Children With Autism Spectrum Disorder (ASD)	13–30 y
NCT04060030[b]	Antioxidant	Treatment of Social and Language Deficits With Leucovorin for Young Children With Autism	**18–54 y**
NCT02677051[b]	Antioxidant	Sulforaphane in a New Jersey (NJ) Population of Individuals With Autism	5–17 y
NCT04060017[b]	Folic acid	Early Treatment of Language Impairment in Young Children With Autism Spectrum Disorder With Leucovorin Calcium	5–12 y
NCT02627508[b]	CB1	Pilot Trial of Pregnenolone in Autism	17–30 y
NCT02649959[c]	Chymotrypsin	An Open Label Study of CM-AT for the Treatment of Children With Autism	8–11 y

(continued on next page)

Table 1 (continued)			
Trial Number	Target	Title	Age Range
NCT03715153[c]	NKCC1	Efficacy and Safety of Bumetanide Oral Liquid Formulation in Children Aged From 2 to <7 Years Old With ASD	5–8 y
NCT03715166[c]	NKCC1	Efficacy and Safety of Bumetanide Oral Liquid Formulation in Children and Adolescents Aged From 7 to <18 Years Old With ASD	6–17 y
Neuropeptides			
NCT02741063[a]	OxtR	Oxytocin Effect on Attentional Bias Toward Emotional Expression Faces in Individuals With High and Low Autistic Traits: (fMRI) Study	**5–40 y**
NCT01931033	OxtR	An Open-Label Trial of Oxytocin in Adolescents With Autism Spectrum Disorders	18–35 y
NCT03293511	OxtR	Oxytocin Modulates Eye Gaze Behavior During Social Processing	5–17 y
NCT02149823[a]	OxtR	Examining Dose-Related Effects of Oxytocin on Social Cognition Across Populations	**18 y and older**
NCT03610919[a]	OxtR	Effects of Oxytocin Dose Frequency on Behavioral and Neural Responses	**16–65 y**
NCT04007224[a]	OxtR	Oxytocin vs Cord Blood for Improving Autistic Disorder	16 y and older
NCT03337035[a]	OxtR	Probiotics and Oxytocin Nasal Spray on Social Behaviors of Autism Spectrum Disorder (ASD) Children	**12–55 y**
NCT04049578[a]	AVPR1a	A Study to Investigate the Pharmacokinetics, Safety, and Tolerability of Balovaptan in Children With Autism Spectrum Disorder	7–24 y
NCT01525901[b]	IGF1R	Clinical Trial in 22q13 Deletion Syndrome(Phelan-McDermid Syndrome)	**18–60 y**
NCT03466671[b]	OxtR	A Trial of TTA-121 on Autism Spectrum Disorder	**18 y and older**
NCT01970345[b]	IGF1R	A Pilot Treatment Study of Insulin-Like Growth Factor-1 (IGF-1) in Autism Spectrum Disorder	3–8 y

(continued on next page)

Table 1 (continued)			
Trial Number	**Target**	**Title**	**Age Range**
NCT02493426[b]	OxtR	Single Dose Intranasal Oxytocin and Cognitive Effects in Autism	2–6 y
NCT02901431[b]	OxtR	A Study to Investigate the Efficacy and Safety of Balovaptan (RO5285119) in Participants With Autism Spectrum Disorder (ASD)	5–12 y
Cannabinoids			
NCT03537950	CB1/CB2	Shifting Brain Excitation-Inhibition Balance in Autism Spectrum Disorder	14–25 y
NCT03664232[b]	FAAH	A Study to Investigate the Efficacy, Safety, and Tolerability of JNJ-42165279 in Adolescent and Adult Participants With ASD	2–6 y
NCT03900923[b]	CB1/CB2	Cannabidiol for ASD Open Trial	7–17 y
NCT03944447[b]	CB1/CB2	Outcomes Mandate National Integration With Cannabis as Medicine	3–17 y
NCT03202303[b]	CB1/CB2	Cannabidivarin (CBDV) vs Placebo in Children With Autism Spectrum Disorder (ASD)	30–60 mo
NCT03849456[b]	CB1/CB2	Safety and Tolerability of Cannabidivarin (CBDV) in Children and Young Adults With Autism Spectrum Disorder	30–60 mo

Bold text indicates studies in adults older than 35 y.
[a] Clinical trial phase: phase 1.
[b] Clinical trial phase: phase 2.
[c] Clinical trial phase: phase 3.

models reflect the complexity associated with excitatory/inhibitory imbalance, despite considerable study.

Glutamate and GABA have been studied in preclinical and human clinical models related to ASD. Genetic research has implicated several genes that encode to proteins on glutamatergic synapses, including SHANK, neurexins, and neuroligins[19]; UBE3A, a gene implicated in Angelman syndrome[20]; and SCN2A, which regulates sodium channels on glutamatergic synapses.[21] Fragile X syndrome (FXS) is the most common single-gene disorder associated with ASD, with deficits noted in the FMR1 gene associated with downregulation of FMRP, a protein that plays a critical role in neurodevelopment including brain growth. Glutamate agonism increases dendritic arborization in wild-type mice, but not ASD FMR1 knock-out mice, suggesting a lack of functioning glutamatergic synapses.[22] Multiple glutamatergic receptors (eg, mGlu5 5, 2, 3, 7) have been implicated in ASD as potential targets for treatment, whereas only one or two have been studied to date with potential drug candidates.[23,24]

Postmortem studies in humans show decreases in glutaminase, a precursor to glutamate in cortical brain regions of individuals with ASD as compared with control subjects,[25] and reduced numbers of GABA receptors in areas relevant to processing of facial information.[26]

Individuals with ASD have a 25% to 30% comorbidity with epilepsy, and GABAergic medicines, such as gabapentin, valproate, and phenobarbital, are used for treatment, although they confer little or no benefit for ASD core symptoms.[27] More recently arbaclofen, a GABA-b agonist, has been tried as a potential treatment of ASD and FXS. Results from several large, placebo-controlled phase 2 trials in FXS[28] and ASD[29] were largely negative for core ASD symptoms. Two additional placebo-controlled studies with arbaclofen in ASD are ongoing to determine if a subset of individuals may be responsive (ClinicalTrials.gov study NCT03682978 and NCT03887676).

Glutamate antagonists have also been studied in ASD and related syndromes, with limited clinical effect. Despite positive results in open-label studies of memantine, an NMDA receptor antagonist, later double-blind placebo-controlled studies were negative for primary and secondary end points.[30] Other compounds, such as acamprosate and amantadine, have been tested in either uncontrolled or small double-blind studies with limited effects.[23] Preclinical ASD models derived from genetic research in FXS demonstrated reversal of decreased glutamatergic signaling with mGlur5 antagonists, leading to several mGlur5 antagonist programs, including basimglurant, fenobam, and mavoglurant. In these studies, most of which were in adolescents and adults, mGlur5 antagonists failed to achieve statistically significant improvements in ASD symptoms.[24] Other NMDA modulators, such as N-acetylcysteine, have been negative for core ASD symptoms.[31] Another compound, riluzole, which is purported to reduce glutamate via sodium channels, was tested in ASD but did not show significant improvement in irritability or core ASD symptoms.[32] Other glutamatergic and GABAergic targets continue to be of interest, although few or no drug candidates have been tested in human trials.[33]

Inflammation and Immunology

Converging evidence suggests that immunologic and inflammatory processes may increase the risk for developing, or may worsen the symptoms of, ASD.[34] Although much of this work is exploratory, data from converging sources have been presented in several recent reviews.[35–37] It is well known that individuals with ASD have higher rates of autoimmune disorders, and increased family history of immune dysfunction.[34] Neuroinflammatory processes, during the prenatal period and early development, confer increased risk for ASD diagnosis or worsening of ASD symptoms, potentially via toxic effects on microglia and astrocytes. These structural effects impact neurotransmission, synaptic plasticity, and other brain functions.[36,38]

Many studies have documented elevated rates of proinflammatory cytokines in individuals with ASD, including plasma tumor necrosis factor-α, interleukin (IL)-1β, IL-6, IL-8, IL-12p40, and others; overproduction of cytokines including interferon-γ and ILs in peripheral blood monocytes[37]; and IL-6 in postmortem brain tissue.[39,40]

Several mechanisms for increased cytokines in ASD have been theorized. Elevated circulating prenatal maternal IgG antibodies or elevated cytokines during gestation[41] are observed in mothers of children who go on to develop ASD. Gastrointestinal hyperpermeability (ie, "leaky gut") and increased levels of harmful gut microbiota have also been postulated as contributing to the proinflammatory cascade.[37] Maternal-fetal inflammation, and subsequent fetal or neonatal inflammatory syndrome, is a hypothesized factor in the increased prevalence of ASD in babies born prematurely.[42] Preclinical models of ASD recapitulate these myriad findings.[43] In addition, purinergic signaling may play a role in neuroinflammation via P2X7, an ion channel regulated by ATP, which could trigger release of proinflammatory cytokines.[44]

Research into potential causative factors has led to testing of treatments that target neuroinflammation, with the goal of improving ASD symptoms, in preclinical models and in humans. Medication studies include cyclooxygenase-2 inhibitors, corticosteroids, and intravenous immunoglobulin: studies are generally small, in combination with other medicines or with usual care, and show limited effect.[43] Antibiotics, such as minocycline, have been studied for symptomatic ASD treatment.[45] Despite little benefit from these early studies, controlled studies are ongoing (NCT04031755). Other experimental treatments have also been studied in open-label trials, such as pentoxifylline,[35] or purinergic compounds, such as suramin[46] (recently completed trial NCT02508259). Newer targets are emerging from this line of research, such as P2X7 antagonists, some of which are already being investigated for efficacy in other conditions, such as depression (NCT04116606).

Neuropeptides

There has been long-standing interest in the closely related neuropeptides oxytocin (OT) and vasopressin (AVP). OT and AVP are cyclic nonapeptides differing in only two amino acids between them, because of sequence similarity in the genes that encode them. Both peptides are synthesized almost exclusively by neurons of the CNS, but act as either neurohormone or neurotransmitter based on differences in their sites of neuronal release. Although the classic hormonal functions of OT on the uterus or AVP (eg, diuresis, vasopressor effects) are the result of release into circulation from nerve terminals in the posterior pituitary, efferent projections from the hypothalamus and amygdala to sites within the CNS give rise a diverse range of effects on behavior, autonomic, and cognitive functions. This partitioning of neurohormonal and neurotransmitter activities is enforced physiologically by the relative impermeability of the blood-brain barrier to the passage of these peptides. OT and AVP have been referred to as yin-yang neuropeptides because of their opposing actions on common neural substrates. A shared family of four G-protein coupled receptors are known to mediate the effects of OT and AVP (AVPR1a, AVPR2, AVPR1b, and OxtR). The OT receptor (OxtR) is the principle receptor for OT throughout the body, and AVPR1a is the most abundantly expressed AVP receptor in the CNS. Both OxtR and AVPR1a have become important targets for medicine development in autism.

OT in particular has been the subject of intense interest from the autism field for more than 20 years. It could be argued that OT has replaced secretin (a gastrointestinal hormone with >15 studies in ASD based on a small case series but proven through large controlled trials to be ineffective[47]) as the most intensely studied therapeutic hypothesis in autism. Much of the interest in OT and autism emerges from work across species establishing a role for central oxytocinergic function in social behavior, including mice, voles, monkeys, and humans. Alterations in plasma OT levels have been reported in ASD,[48] including correlations with symptom severity[49] and evidence of disrupted processing of active OT peptide from its genetically encoded precursor.[50] Genetic variants in the human OxtR gene have also frequently been associated with ASD,[51] with evidence pointing to a relationship between OxtR genotype in OT efficacy in clinical studies.[52] Collectively, the directionality of evidence has consistently implicated OxtR agonists (or PAMs) as a desired pharmacologic profile. This has been corroborated by work with synthetic OT in preclinical models of ASD. For example, OT attenuates social interaction deficits in the valproate paradigm.[53] In BALB/cByJ and C58/J mice, both inbred strain models of ASD, OT reverses social deficits and exhibited efficacy with repetitive behaviors.[54,55] Numerous experimental medicine studies in humans have taken advantage of widely available synthetic OT to investigate the translatability of efficacy observed in animal models to ASD patients. Collectively, the evidence from animal models to human ASD consistently points to a role for central oxytocinergic function in regulating social deficits ASD, and points to OxtR agonism, or positive allosteric modulation of OxtR function as an attractive target concept for ASD therapeutics development, with particular relevance to social deficits and social anxiety.

Similar to OT, a critical role for AVP, and its principle CNS receptor AVPR1a, in the regulation of social behavior has been established in numerous mammalian species.[56,57] Collectively, the available evidence has pointed to antagonism, or negative allosteric modulation, of AVPR1a as a plausible mechanistic hypothesis for therapeutics development in ASD. Indeed, this has inspired the discovery and development of molecules based on this mechanism of action, as exemplified by the selective AVPR1a antagonist balovaptan (RO5285119), which recently advanced to phase 3 (NCT03504917) as an experimental therapeutic for ASD.

Melanocortin is another neuropeptide implicated in ASD. MCR4 is a family of four GPCRs responsible for mediating the biologic effects of α-melanocyte-stimulating hormone, a peptide derived from the enzymatic processing of pro-opiomelanocortin in mammals. Evidence suggests that the effects of MC4R agonism on social behaviors relevant to autism are the result of its stimulatory effects on central oxytocinergic activity. MC4R agonism leads to release of OT, increased brain levels of OT levels, and increased prosocial behavior. In the $Cntnap3^{-/-}$ mouse model of autism, which is hallmarked by deficits in social behavior and reduced central oxytocinergic tone (decreased cerebrospinal fluid levels of peptide and number of OT-positive neurons in the paraventricular nucleus of the hypothalamus), the selective MC4R agonist melanotan-II rescues the social abnormalities and these effects are blocked by cotreatment with an OxtR antagonist.[58] Interest in MC4R as a possible target for therapeutics development in autism is further supported by evidence of prosocial efficacy in other preclinical models of autism. The maternal immune activation paradigm in mice is a commonly used preclinical paradigm to assess potential efficacy of experimental therapeutics for ASD.[59] In the maternal immune activation paradigm, melanotan-II selectively improves social deficits without impacting similar behaviors in unaffected animals.[60] Based on the evidence to date, MC4R has emerged as a target of interest in addressing the core social domains for ASD.

Endocannabinoids

The endocannabinoid system, including the cannabinoid receptor 1 and 2 (CB1, CB2), the fatty acid amides, N-arachidonoylethanolamine, or anandamide (AEA) and 2-arachidonoyl-sn-glycerol and their associated synthetic and catabolic enzymes is believed to play important roles in the regulation of the immune system, pain perception, affect, motivation, emotion, fear and anxiety responses. Evidence has demonstrated that the endocannabinoid system is involved in behavior and emotion directly relevant to ASD.[61] Anecdotal evidence from the use of cannabis and its derivatives by people with ASD suggests beneficial effects on the core symptoms of ASD.

Results from preclinical and clinical studies on ASD have determined that variation and disruption of the endocannabinoid system are associated with behavioral and biomarker changes.[61–63] Specifically, the CB1 cannabinoid receptors and their endogenous ligands (AEA and 2-arachidonoyl-sn-glycerol) have been associated with modulating social play and social anxiety, two pivotal facets of social behavior.[64–67] In a study that examined genes with abnormal expression levels in the cerebella of subjects with autism compared with control subjects, it was determined that the CB_1 gene demonstrated a 30% downregulation in subjects with autism.[68] Furthermore, CB_1 gene variations contributed to regulating the perception of signals of social reward, such as happy faces, suggesting that CB_1 is a critical component in the molecular perception of social behavior.[69] Circulating levels of AEA have been found to be lower in children with ASD.[70,71]

Inhibitors of fatty acid amide hydrolase, the main degradative enzyme of AEA, and other endocannabinoid modulators reverse core ASD behaviors and comorbidities in various preclinical models.[39,72–76] In addition, heightened AEA signaling (via fatty acid amide hydrolase inhibition) stimulates social reward and occludes the prosocial effects of OT, suggesting OT's effects may be at least partially mediated through the endocannabinoid system.[77–79] Several clinical trials testing modulation of the endocannabinoid system in ASD either by administration of cannabinoids or by inhibition of endocannabinoid degrading enzymes have been completed or are underway. A randomized, placebo-controlled study testing a cannabidiol/tetrahydrocannabinol (two cannabinoids present in cannabis) mixture in 150 children showed promising results.[80] Six ongoing studies are listed in **Table 1**.

Channelopathies

Combined advances in genomic sequencing technologies and large-scale digital phenotyping cohorts have given rise to an unprecedented growth in the understanding of the complex genetic risk architecture underlying ASD. Pathogenic variation in genes encoding ion channels have become common in the expanding genomic map of syndromic causes of ASD. From a drug development perspective, ion channels are widely embraced as a precedented ("drugable") class of molecular targets given the extensive number of marketed medicines that work through the modulation of channel function.[81] This is especially true in the context of CNS drug discovery, and collectively has provided the unmet medical needs of the ASD field with opportunities to leverage extensive prior experience and know-how working with familiar channel targets newly implicated with ASD through genomics.

Although ASD-related channelopathies have been described among the ligand-gated family of channels modulated by the amino acid neurotransmitters GABA and glutamate, because these have been addressed previously, we focus on channel targets and channelopathies involved in voltage-gated, and/or calcium-activated, conductance of potassium (K^+), sodium (Na^+), and calcium (Ca^{+2}) across cellular membranes. Our use of the term "channelopathy" here simply refers to a biologic state created by the loss or gain of a specific channel's function, which in most cases referenced here are the result of pathogenic variation in the gene encoding that channel. In most cases these mutations result in characteristically a clinical phenotype or syndrome. A channelopathy may also arise as a consequence of interactions with a disease process or pathobiology. Across these examples we have attempted to focus attention onto channels that represent promising targets for therapeutics development in ASD.

Timothy syndrome is caused by pathogenic mutations in the *CACNA1C* gene, which encodes the voltage-dependent calcium channel $Ca_V1.2$. Timothy syndrome is an autosomal-dominant syndrome characterized clinically by the presence of prolonged ventricular repolarization and a cardiac arrhythmia syndrome long QT. Dysmorphic facial features, seizures, and hypotonia are also part of the clinical construct, in addition to an ASD prevalence estimated to be as high as 80%.[82] $Ca_V1.2$ is a member of the L-type calcium channel family that industry has had prior success developing blockers and openers against.

Several channelopathies have been directly implicated in the underlying pathophysiology of FXS because of their functional interactions with the fragile X mental retardation protein (FMRP). Genetic loss of FMRP expression is the primary cause of FXS. In addition to its well-known RNA-binding functions, FMRP also directly interacts with ion channels to regulate synaptic function across the CNS.[83] Among FMRP's ion channel targets is Kv3.1 (Slack channels), a potassium channel directly linked to sensory hypersensitivities and cognitive deficits in FXS.[84] In the *Fmr1-/y* genetic mouse model of FXS, positive modulators of Kv3.1/3.2 channels demonstrated the ability to rescue sensory processing abnormalities, implicating these channels as target for potential therapeutics development.[85] Building off this, Autifony Therapeutics has already been granted an Orphan Designation by the Food and Drug Administration for their Kv3.1 modulator AUT00206 in FXS.

Like Kv3.1/Slack channels, another potassium channel target of FMRP has been implicated as a putative target for therapeutics development in FXS. This target, the so-called "big potassium" (BK) channels (Maxi-K, Slo1, Cav1.1), are unique in their sensitivity to calcium (Ca^{+2}) and voltage, and by a massive conductance of potassium by the channel when activated. Like Slack channels, BK is a known target of FMRP function, which regulates BK channel Ca^{+2} sensitivity through interactions with the channel's Beta4 subunit.[86] Targeting BK channels as a therapeutic approach in FXS has strong support from extensive preclinical profiling of the BK channel opener compounds, such as BMS-204352 in *Fmr1-/y* mice mouse model of FXS, where it shows a broad range of efficacies on cognition, hyperactivity, and autism-like phenotypes (repetitive behaviors and social behavior).[87,88]

In Pitt-Hopkins syndrome (PTHS), a rare genetic syndrome and known cause of ASD, recent interest has fallen on the sodium channel. PTHS is caused by mutations in transcription factor 4 (TCF4), which is key for this and that. In PTHS, the increased expression of SCN10 AM (NaV1.8) and KCNQ1 implicates a combined channelopathy at the endophenotypic center of this rare ASD.[89,90] Because NaV1.8 has been a high-interest target of the pain field for several years, the PTHS field has already begun to take advantage of compounds developed to target this channel as experimental analgesics to help expand the validity of this target for PTHS, ASD, and related indications.[91]

Other Targets of Interest

Several other approaches are under consideration, or early study, for efficacy in the treatment of ASD. Stem cell treatments of various types are currently being evaluated in several trials under the hypothesis that the various trophic factors secreted may positively affect several of the systems discussed previously.[92,93] Fecal transplants and probiotics are also being studied based on the well-known presence of gut abnormalities in children with ASD.[94] Another interesting approach stems from the observation that ASD symptoms seem to improve in the presence of fever.[95] Thus, approaches to safely mimic the effects of fever are being considered. Finally, nutritional insufficiencies are widely recognized in some individuals with ASD and medical foods or nutritional supplementation may have the potential to impact this insufficiency and several of the mechanisms we have described previously.[96]

SUMMARY AND CHALLENGES FOR THE DEVELOPMENT OF PHARMACOLOGIC TREATMENTS ACROSS THE AGE RANGE

Although clinical trial results from pharmacologic treatments of ASD thus far show promise, results remain highly variable in treatment of core symptoms, and there is yet to be a robust demonstration of efficacy that would implicate one or more pathways or targets for one treatment over another.

In designing a drug development plan for a treatment of the core symptoms of ASD it is critical to account for the fact that ASD is a neurodevelopmental disorder spanning the full human lifespan, and that efficacy and response to specific treatments may differ across that span. Studies have consistently demonstrated age-dependent changes in the prevalence of psychotropic medication use.[97] Although there are still questions about the hierarchy of evidence supporting the safety and efficacy of such use, it is clear that the unmet clinical needs of individuals with ASD change across the lifespan, which suggests that relevance of specific classes of new (experimental) or older medicines (and the molecular targets through which they act) may also vary across the lifespan. One cannot assume that the biology engaged by new, diverse targets will be consistent throughout all phases of development. It is therefore reasonable that initial approval for an ASD treatment would include children and young adults. Analogies can be drawn to attention-deficit/hyperactivity disorder where the Food and Drug Administration requires initial new drug applications to include children down to 6 years of age. As part of the drug development it is likely that distinct clinical trials in children and adults would be necessary to ensure efficacy and safety in both groups. After initial approval younger and older individuals with ASD could be studied as part of postapproval commitment, or via other mechanisms.

In addition, although there is reason to be optimistic that many of the drug targets discussed here offer opportunities to reduce the clinical burden of specific symptoms in an acute setting (eg, anxiety, seizure, sleep), it must be assumed that ability to address and improve an individual's autism cannot occur with pharmacologic treatment alone. It must work in conjunction with the current standards of care (eg, behavioral interventions, cognitive behavioral, occupational, and speech therapies) to improve outcomes over the lifespan. Understanding and optimizing these adjunctive interactions will remain a challenge for the field.

A further challenge in development of psychopharmacologic treatment in ASD stems from the lack of validated research end points. In contrast to more mature areas of medicine development in psychiatry and neurology, where there is an abundance of regulatory precedence in terms of end points and other measures of clinical outcome, the ASD space is still early as a therapeutic area of interest. Developmental changes and heterogeneity of symptoms further add to the challenge in identifying suitable outcome measures. That said, there have been significant innovations in the area of end point development. For example, the Autism Behavior Inventory[98] and the Autism Impact Measure[99] are two caregiver-reported outcome measures that have been specifically developed to measure change in symptoms in ASD in the context of treatment trials. The Autism Impact Measure is suitable for children only, whereas the Autism Behavior Inventory has been validated in children and adult ASD populations. In addition, international consortiums and pharmacologic companies are working to develop technological applications that may lead to the development of more objective end points and biomarkers for ASD (EU AIMS-2: children, adolescents, and adults [https://www.aims-2-trials.eu]; ABC-CT: children and adolescents [https://fnih.org/what-we-do/biomarkers-consortium/programs/autism-biomarkers]).[100]

Finally, several brain pathways and neurobiologic systems have been identified as potentially involved in the development and maintenance of ASD symptoms. Although there may be common brain pathways resulting in similar phenotypic presentation, there are also likely to be subtypes of ASD resulting from different biologic underpinnings, as is evident from rare genetic disorders with high comorbidity with ASD, such as Phelan McDermid syndrome, or FXS. Additionally, these different groups will be variable in terms of the course of development, comorbidities, and response to treatment. Because of this heterogeneity, the wide variety of targets, and the current lack of clarity as to the best approaches for measurement of outcomes, a platform study design may be ideal at the proof of concept stage. Platform trials use adaptive outcomes designs to simultaneously investigate multiple treatments. Such a study could allow several compounds to be tested efficiently (simultaneously, or in an ongoing, rolling fashion) within the framework of a single study, sharing a single infrastructure and potentially created by a public-private partnership collaboration.

The wealth of new data generated in genetic research and the growth of small biotechnology companies and efforts around identification of autism biomarkers for clinical trials is leading to a host of promising new targets with the potential to improve the lives of individuals with autism.

DISCLOSURE STATEMENT

R.H. Ring works for a company involved in the discovery and development of therapeutics for genetic syndromes that cause autism. The company is a research company and has no commercial products of any kind. G. Pandina, A. Bangerter, and S. Ness are full-time employees and stockholders at Janssen Research & Development, LLC.

REFERENCES

1. Bal VH, Kim SH, Fok M, et al. Autism spectrum disorder symptoms from ages 2 to 19 years: implications for diagnosing adolescents and young adults. Autism Res 2019;12(1):89–99.
2. Siebes R, Muntjewerff J-W, Staal W. Differences of symptom distribution across adult age in high functioning individuals on the autism spectrum using sub-scales of the autism spectrum quotient. J Autism Dev Disord 2018;48(11): 3939–44.
3. Piven J, Harper J, Palmer P, et al. Course of behavioral change in autism: a retrospective study of high-IQ adolescents and adults. J Am Acad Child Adolesc Psychiatry 1996;35(4):523–9.
4. Seltzer MM, Krauss MW, Shattuck PT, et al. The symptoms of autism spectrum disorders in adolescence and adulthood. J Autism Dev Disord 2003;33(6): 565–81.
5. Shattuck PT, Seltzer MM, Greenberg JS, et al. Change in autism symptoms and maladaptive behaviors in adolescents and adults with an autism spectrum disorder. J Autism Dev Disord 2007;37(9):1735–47.
6. Magiati I, Tay XW, Howlin P. Cognitive, language, social and behavioural outcomes in adults with autism spectrum disorders: a systematic review of longitudinal follow-up studies in adulthood. Clin Psychol Rev 2014;34(1):73–86.
7. Esbensen AJ, Seltzer MM, Lam KS, et al. Age-related differences in restricted repetitive behaviors in autism spectrum disorders. J Autism Dev Disord 2009; 39(1):57–66.
8. Howlin P, Savage S, Moss P, et al. Cognitive and language skills in adults with autism: a 40-year follow-up. J Child Psychol Psychiatry 2014;55(1):49–58.
9. Militerni R, Bravaccio C, Falco C, et al. Repetitive behaviors in autistic disorder. Eur Child Adolesc Psychiatry 2002;11(5):210–8.
10. Gillespie-Lynch K, Sepeta L, Wang Y, et al. Early childhood predictors of the social competence of adults with autism. J Autism Dev Disord 2012;42(2):161–74.
11. McGovern CW, Sigman M. Continuity and change from early childhood to adolescence in autism. J Child Psychol Psychiatry 2005;46(4):401–8.
12. Billstedt E, Carina Gillberg I, Gillberg C. Autism in adults: symptom patterns and early childhood predictors. Use of the DISCO in a community sample followed from childhood. J Child Psychol Psychiatry 2007;48(11):1102–10.
13. Taylor JL, Seltzer MM. Changes in the autism behavioral phenotype during the transition to adulthood. J Autism Dev Disord 2010;40(12):1431–46.

14. Dawson G, Burner K. Behavioral interventions in children and adolescents with autism spectrum disorder: a review of recent findings. Curr Opin Pediatr 2011; 23(6):616–20.

15. Aman MG, Mcdougle CJ, Scahill L, et al. Medication and parent training in children with pervasive developmental disorders and serious behavior problems: results from a randomized clinical trial. J Am Acad Child Adolesc Psychiatry 2009;48(12):1143–54.

16. Jobski K, Höfer J, Hoffmann F, et al. Use of psychotropic drugs in patients with autism spectrum disorders: a systematic review. Acta Psychiatr Scand 2017; 135(1):8–28.

17. Howes OD, Rogdaki M, Findon JL, et al. Autism spectrum disorder: consensus guidelines on assessment, treatment and research from the British Association for Psychopharmacology. J Psychopharmacol 2018;32(1):3–29.

18. Uzunova G, Pallanti S, Hollander E. Excitatory/inhibitory imbalance in autism spectrum disorders: implications for interventions and therapeutics. World J Biol Psychiatry 2016;17(3):174–86.

19. Chen J, Yu S, Fu Y, et al. Synaptic proteins and receptors defects in autism spectrum disorders. Front Cell Neurosci 2014;8:276.

20. Sonzogni M, Hakonen J, Kleijn MB, et al. Delayed loss of UBE3A reduces the expression of Angelman syndrome-associated phenotypes. Mol Autism 2019; 10(1):23.

21. Spratt PW, Ben-Shalom R, Keeshen CM, et al. The autism-associated gene Scn2a contributes to dendritic excitability and synaptic function in the prefrontal cortex. Neuron 2019;103(4):673–85.e5.

22. Cruz-Martín A, Crespo M, Portera-Cailliau C. Glutamate induces the elongation of early dendritic protrusions via mGluRs in wild type mice, but not in fragile X mice. PLoS One 2012;7(2):e32446.

23. Rojas DC. The role of glutamate and its receptors in autism and the use of glutamate receptor antagonists in treatment. J Neural Transm 2014;121(8):891–905.

24. Erickson CA, Davenport MH, Schaefer TL, et al. Fragile X targeted pharmacotherapy: lessons learned and future directions. J Neurodev Disord 2017;9(1):7.

25. Shimmura C, Suzuki K, Iwata Y, et al. Enzymes in the glutamate-glutamine cycle in the anterior cingulate cortex in postmortem brain of subjects with autism. Mol Autism 2013;4(1):6.

26. Oblak AL, Gibbs TT, Blatt GJ. Reduced GABAA receptors and benzodiazepine binding sites in the posterior cingulate cortex and fusiform gyrus in autism. Brain Res 2011;1380:218–28.

27. Frye RE, Rossignol D, Casanova MF, et al. A review of traditional and novel treatments for seizures in autism spectrum disorder: findings from a systematic review and expert panel. Front Public Health 2013;1:31.

28. Berry-Kravis E, Hagerman R, Visootsak J, et al. Arbaclofen in fragile X syndrome: results of phase 3 trials. J Neurodev Disord 2017;9(1):3.

29. Veenstra-VanderWeele J, Cook EH, King BH, et al. Arbaclofen in children and adolescents with autism spectrum disorder: a randomized, controlled, phase 2 trial. Neuropsychopharmacology 2017;42(7):1390.

30. Hardan AY, Hendren RL, Aman MG, et al. Efficacy and safety of memantine in children with autism spectrum disorder: results from three phase 2 multicenter studies. Autism 2019;23(8):2096–111.

31. Goel R, Hong JS, Findling RL, et al. An update on pharmacotherapy of autism spectrum disorder in children and adolescents. Int Rev Psychiatry 2018;30(1): 78–95.

32. De Boer J, Vingerhoets C, Hirdes M, et al. Efficacy and tolerability of riluzole in psychiatric disorders: a systematic review and preliminary meta-analysis. Psychiatry Res 2019;278:294–302.

33. Lacivita E, Perrone R, Margari L, et al. Targets for drug therapy for autism spectrum disorder: challenges and future directions. J Med Chem 2017;60(22): 9114–41.

34. Thom RP, Keary CJ, Palumbo ML, et al. Beyond the brain: a multi-system inflammatory subtype of autism spectrum disorder. Psychopharmacology (Berl) 2019; 236(10):3045–61.

35. Marchezan J, dos Santos EGAW, Deckmann I, et al. Immunological dysfunction in autism spectrum disorder: a potential target for therapy. Neuroimmunomodulation 2018;25(5–6):300–19.

36. Matta SM, Hill-Yardin EL, Crack PJ. The influence of neuroinflammation in autism spectrum disorder. Brain Behav Immun 2019;79:75–90.

37. Siniscalco D, Schultz S, Brigida AL, et al. Inflammation and neuro-immune dysregulations in autism spectrum disorders. Pharmaceuticals 2018;11(2):56.

38. Petrelli F, Pucci L, Bezzi P. Astrocytes and microglia and their potential link with autism spectrum disorders. Front Cell Neurosci 2016;10:21.

39. Wu H-F, Lu T-Y, Chu M-C, et al. Targeting the inhibition of fatty acid amide hydrolase ameliorate the endocannabinoid-mediated synaptic dysfunction in a valproic acid-induced rat model of autism. Neuropharmacology 2019;162:107736.

40. Vargas DL, Nascimbene C, Krishnan C, et al. Neuroglial activation and neuroinflammation in the brain of patients with autism. Ann Neurol 2005;57(1):67–81.

41. Meltzer A, Van de Water J. The role of the immune system in autism spectrum disorder. Neuropsychopharmacology 2017;42(1):284.

42. Bokobza C, Van Steenwinckel J, Mani S, et al. Neuroinflammation in preterm babies and autism spectrum disorders. Pediatr Res 2019;85(2):155–65.

43. McDougle CJ, Landino SM, Vahabzadeh A, et al. Toward an immune-mediated subtype of autism spectrum disorder. Brain Res 2015;1617:72–92.

44. Bhattacharya A, Biber K. The microglial ATP-gated ion channel P2X7 as a CNS drug target. Glia 2016;64(10):1772–87.

45. Pardo CA, Buckley A, Thurm A, et al. A pilot open-label trial of minocycline in patients with autism and regressive features. J Neurodev Disord 2013;5(1):9.

46. Naviaux RK, Curtis B, Li K, et al. Low-dose suramin in autism spectrum disorder: a small, phase I/II, randomized clinical trial. Ann Clin Transl Neurol 2017;4(7): 491–505.

47. Williams K, Wray JA, Wheeler DM. Intravenous secretin for autism spectrum disorders (ASD). Cochrane Database Syst Rev 2012;(4):CD003495.

48. Taurines R, Schwenck C, Lyttwin B, et al. Oxytocin plasma concentrations in children and adolescents with autism spectrum disorder: correlation with autistic symptomatology. Atten Defic Hyperact Disord 2014;6(3):231–9.

49. Kobylinska L, Panaitescu AM, Gabreanu G, et al. Plasmatic levels of neuropeptides, including oxytocin, in children with autism spectrum disorder, correlate with the disorder severity. Acta Endocrinol (Buchar) 2019;5(1):16–24.

50. Green L, Fein D, Modahl C, et al. Oxytocin and autistic disorder: alterations in peptide forms. Biol Psychiatry 2001;50(8):609–13.

51. LoParo D, Waldman ID. The oxytocin receptor gene (OXTR) is associated with autism spectrum disorder: a meta-analysis. Mol Psychiatry 2015;20(5):640–6.

52. Kosaka H, Okamoto Y, Munesue T, et al. Oxytocin efficacy is modulated by dosage and oxytocin receptor genotype in young adults with high-functioning autism: a 24-week randomized clinical trial. Transl Psychiatry 2016;6(8):e872.

53. Hara Y, Ago Y, Higuchi M, et al. Oxytocin attenuates deficits in social interaction but not recognition memory in a prenatal valproic acid-induced mouse model of autism. Horm Behav 2017;96:130–6.

54. Teng BL, Nonneman RJ, Agster KL, et al. Prosocial effects of oxytocin in two mouse models of autism spectrum disorders. Neuropharmacology 2013;72: 187–96.

55. Teng BL, Nikolova VD, Riddick NV, et al. Reversal of social deficits by sub-chronic oxytocin in two autism mouse models. Neuropharmacology 2016;105: 61–71.

56. Charles R, Sakurai T, Takahashi N, et al. Introduction of the human AVPR1A gene substantially alters brain receptor expression patterns and enhances aspects of social behavior in transgenic mice. Dis Model Mech 2014;7(8):1013–22.

57. Goodson JL, Bass AH. Social behavior functions and related anatomical characteristics of vasotocin/vasopressin systems in vertebrates. Brain Res Brain Res Rev 2001;35(3):246–65.

58. Penagarikano O, Lazaro MT, Lu XH, et al. Exogenous and evoked oxytocin restores social behavior in the Cntnap2 mouse model of autism. Sci Transl Med 2015;7(271):271ra278.

59. Lammert CR, Lukens JR. Modeling autism-related disorders in mice with maternal immune activation (MIA). Methods Mol Biol 2019;1960:227–36.

60. Minakova E, Lang J, Medel-Matus JS, et al. Melanotan-II reverses autistic features in a maternal immune activation mouse model of autism. PLoS One 2019;14(1):e0210389.

61. Solinas M, Goldberg SR, Piomelli D. The endocannabinoid system in brain reward processes. Br J Pharmacol 2008;154(2):369–83.

62. Fletcher P, Shallice T, Dolan RJ. The functional roles of prefrontal cortex in episodic memory. I. Encoding. Brain 1998;121(7):1239–48.

63. Smith DR, Stanley CM, Foss T, et al. Rare genetic variants in the endocannabinoid system genes CNR1 and DAGLA are associated with neurological phenotypes in humans. PLoS One 2017;12(11):e0187926.

64. Pacey A, Povey A, Clyma J-A, et al. Modifiable and non-modifiable risk factors for poor sperm morphology. Hum Reprod 2014;29(8):1629–36.

65. Stel M, van den Heuvel C, Smeets RC. Facial feedback mechanisms in autistic spectrum disorders. J Autism Dev Disord 2008;38(7):1250–8.

66. Földy C, Malenka RC, Südhof TC. Autism-associated neuroligin-3 mutations commonly disrupt tonic endocannabinoid signaling. Neuron 2013;78(3): 498–509.

67. Battista N, Meccariello R, Cobellis G, et al. The role of endocannabinoids in gonadal function and fertility along the evolutionary axis. Mol Cell Endocrinol 2012;355(1):1–14.

68. Paul R, Chawarska K, Fowler C, et al. "Listen my children and you shall hear": auditory preferences in toddlers with autism spectrum disorders. J Speech Lang Hear Res 2007;50(5):1350–64.

69. Burnham D, Dodd B. Auditory–visual speech integration by prelinguistic infants: perception of an emergent consonant in the McGurk effect. Dev Psychobiol 2004;45(4):204–20.

70. Aran A, Eylon M, Harel M, et al. Lower circulating endocannabinoid levels in children with autism spectrum disorder. Mol Autism 2019;10(1):2.

71. Karhson DS, Krasinska KM, Dallaire JA, et al. Plasma anandamide concentrations are lower in children with autism spectrum disorder. Mol Autism 2018; 9(1):18.

72. Kerr D, Downey L, Conboy M, et al. Alterations in the endocannabinoid system in the rat valproic acid model of autism. Behav Brain Res 2013;249:124–32.

73. Trezza V, Vanderschuren LJ. Bidirectional cannabinoid modulation of social behavior in adolescent rats. Psychopharmacology 2008;197(2):217–27.

74. Zamberletti E, Gabaglio M, Woolley-Roberts M, et al. Cannabidivarin treatment ameliorates autism-like behaviors and restores hippocampal endocannabinoid system and glia alterations induced by prenatal valproic acid exposure in rats. Front Cell Neurosci 2019;13:367.

75. Servadio M, Melancia F, Manduca A, et al. Targeting anandamide metabolism rescues core and associated autistic-like symptoms in rats prenatally exposed to valproic acid. Transl Psychiatry 2016;6(9):e902.

76. Doenni V, Gray J, Song C, et al. Deficient adolescent social behavior following early-life inflammation is ameliorated by augmentation of anandamide signaling. Brain Behav Immun 2016;58:237–47.

77. Wei D, Dinh D, Lee D, et al. Enhancement of anandamide-mediated endocannabinoid signaling corrects autism-related social impairment. Cannabis Cannabinoid Res 2016;1(1):81–9.

78. Wei D, Lee D, Cox CD, et al. Endocannabinoid signaling mediates oxytocin-driven social reward. Proc Natl Acad Sci U S A 2015;112(45):14084–9.

79. Wei H, Zou H, Sheikh AM, et al. IL-6 is increased in the cerebellum of autistic brain and alters neural cell adhesion, migration and synaptic formation. J Neuroinflammation 2011;8(1):52.

80. Aran A, Harel M, Polyansky L, et al. A Placebo-controlled trial of cannabinoids in children with ASD. INSAR 2019 Palais des congres de Montreal, May 2, 2019.

81. Gerlach AC, Antonio BM. Validation of ion channel targets. Channels (Austin) 2015;9(6):376–9.

82. Splawski I, Timothy KW, Sharpe LM, et al. Ca(V)1.2 calcium channel dysfunction causes a multisystem disorder including arrhythmia and autism. Cell 2004; 119(1):19–31.

83. Ferron L. Fragile X mental retardation protein controls ion channel expression and activity. J Physiol 2016;594(20):5861–7.

84. Strumbos JG, Brown MR, Kronengold J, et al. Fragile X mental retardation protein is required for rapid experience-dependent regulation of the potassium channel Kv3.1b. J Neurosci 2010;30(31):10263–71.

85. El-Hassar L, Song L, Tan WJT, et al. Modulators of Kv3 potassium channels rescue the auditory function of fragile X mice. J Neurosci 2019;39(24):4797–813.

86. Deng PY, Rotman Z, Blundon JA, et al. FMRP regulates neurotransmitter release and synaptic information transmission by modulating action potential duration via BK channels. Neuron 2013;77(4):696–711.

87. Hebert B, Pietropaolo S, Meme S, et al. Rescue of fragile X syndrome phenotypes in Fmr1 KO mice by a BKCa channel opener molecule. Orphanet J Rare Dis 2014;9:124.

88. Carreno-Munoz MI, Martins F, Medrano MC, et al. Potential involvement of impaired BKCa channel function in sensory defensiveness and some behavioral disturbances induced by unfamiliar environment in a mouse model of fragile X syndrome. Neuropsychopharmacology 2018;43(3):492–502.

89. Rannals MD, Hamersky GR, Page SC, et al. Psychiatric risk gene transcription factor 4 regulates intrinsic excitability of prefrontal neurons via repression of SCN10a and KCNQ1. Neuron 2016;90(1):43–55.

90. Rannals MD, Page SC, Campbell MN, et al. Neurodevelopmental models of transcription factor 4 deficiency converge on a common ion channel as a potential therapeutic target for Pitt Hopkins syndrome. Rare Dis 2016;4(1):e1220468.

91. Ekins S, Gerlach J, Zorn KM, et al. Repurposing approved drugs as inhibitors of Kv7.1 and Nav1.8 to treat Pitt Hopkins syndrome. Pharm Res 2019;36(9):137.

92. Riordan NH, Hincapié ML, Morales I, et al. Allogeneic human umbilical cord mesenchymal stem cells for the treatment of autism spectrum disorder in children: safety profile and effect on cytokine levels. Stem Cells Transl Med 2019; 8(10):1008–16.

93. Carpenter KL, Major S, Tallman C, et al. White matter tract changes associated with clinical improvement in an open-label trial assessing autologous umbilical cord blood for treatment of young children with autism. Stem Cells Transl Med 2019;8(2):138–47.

94. Kang D-W, Adams JB, Coleman DM, et al. Long-term benefit of microbiota transfer therapy on autism symptoms and gut microbiota. Sci Rep 2019;9(1): 5821.

95. Grzadzinski R, Lord C, Sanders SJ, et al. Children with autism spectrum disorder who improve with fever: insights from the Simons Simplex Collection. Autism Res 2018;11(1):175–84.

96. Esteban-Figuerola P, Canals J, Fernández-Cao JC, et al. Differences in food consumption and nutritional intake between children with autism spectrum disorders and typically developing children: a meta-analysis. Autism 2019;23(5): 1079–95.

97. Rasmussen L, Bilenberg N, Thomsen Ernst M, et al. Use of psychotropic drugs among children and adolescents with autism spectrum disorders in Denmark: a nationwide drug utilization study. J Clin Med 2018;7(10) [pii:E339].

98. Bangerter A, Ness S, Lewin D, et al. Clinical validation of the autism behavior inventory: caregiver-rated assessment of core and associated symptoms of autism spectrum disorder. J Autism Dev Disord 2019;1–12. https://doi.org/10. 1007/s10803-019-03965-7.

99. Houghton R, Monz B, Law K, et al. Psychometric validation of the autism impact measure (AIM). J Autism Dev Disord 2019;49(6):2559–70.

100. Ness SL, Manyakov NV, Bangerter A, et al. JAKE® multimodal data capture system: insights from an observational study of autism spectrum disorder. Front Neurosci 2017;11:517.

Autism and Education

Kathleen A. Flannery, MEd[a], Robert Wisner-Carlson, MD[b],*

KEYWORDS

- Autism spectrum disorders • Education • Evidence-based practices • Instruction
- Special education

KEY POINTS

- Special education laws and reform effectuated how individuals with disabilities are educated in the school setting. The Education for All Handicapped Children Act and the Individuals with Disabilities Education Act brought about major requirements, such as individualized education plans, provision of free and appropriate public education, and educating students with disabilities in a least restrictive environment.
- Research identifies specific evidence-based practices as strategies that, when implemented with fidelity, yield successful outcomes for individuals with autism spectrum disorder (ASD) in the school setting. Organizations, such as the National Autism Center and the National Professional Development Center on Autism Spectrum Disorder, provide information and resources on effective evidence-based practices for educating children and youth with ASD.
- Training and preparation for teachers are essential to the education of students with autism. Knowledge of the characteristics of the disorder, possible comorbid factors, best practices, and the unique strengths and difficulties of each student is vital to successful school outcomes for students with autism.
- The transition from high school to postsecondary years is a difficult time for youth with autism. Entitlement services drop off. Therefore, transition planning during the high school years and a strong partnership between the school and family are imperative.

INTRODUCTION

Special education programs did not always exist in the United States. Prior to Supreme Court cases, such as Brown v Board of Education (1954) or PARC v Pennsylvania (1971), and the enactment of the Education for All Handicapped Children Act in 1975, it was common for children with disabilities to be excluded from public school education or receive unequal treatment within the public school system.[1] One of the earliest accounts of an individual being excluded from a public school education dates

---

[a] Sheppard Pratt Health System, 6501 North Charles Street, Towson, MD 21204, USA;
[b] Neuropsychiatry Outpatient Program, Adult Developmental Neuropsychiatry Clinic, Adult Inpatient Intellectual Disability and Autism Unit, Sheppard Pratt Autism Registry, Ethics Committee, Sheppard Pratt Hospital, 6501 North Charles Street, Baltimore, MD 21285, USA
* Corresponding author.
E-mail address: RWisner-Carlson@sheppardpratt.org

Child Adolesc Psychiatric Clin N Am 29 (2020) 319–343
https://doi.org/10.1016/j.chc.2019.12.005   **childpsych.theclinics.com**
1056-4993/20/© 2020 Elsevier Inc. All rights reserved.

to 1893. "In the case of Watson vs. the City of Cambridge, the Massachusetts Supreme Court ruled that a child who was 'weak of mind' and could not benefit from instruction, was troublesome to other children, made 'unusual noises,' and was unable to take 'ordinary, decent, physical care of himself' could be expelled from public school."[2] In 1919, the Wisconsin Supreme Court approved the exclusion of a rising sixth-grade student who was capable of benefiting from public school education but displayed distorted facial features, frequently drooled, and had a speech disorder.[3]

Students diagnosed with autism spectrum disorders (ASDs) may exhibit the characteristics described previously (ie, "weak of mind," "troublesome to other children," "produce unusual noises," and "frequent drooling").[2] In *Thinking in Pictures: My Life with Autism*,[4] Temple Grandin states, "The word 'autism' still conveys a fixed and dreadful meaning to most people—they visualize a child mute, rocking, screaming, inaccessible, cut off from human contact. And we almost always speak of autistic children, never of autistic adults, as if such children never grew up, or were somehow mysteriously spirited off the planet, out of society."[4]

In 2013, the *Diagnostic and Statistical Manual of Mental Disorders, Fifth Edition*,[5] adopted ASD because it is "broadly considered to be a multi-factorial disorder"[6] with a "dyadic definition of core symptoms." Autism is now better defined as a spectrum of disorders that vary in onset, severity of symptoms, and comorbidity.[6]

Autism is a complex, neurodevelopmental disorder that is characterized by impairments in communication and social interaction combined with repetitive or rigid behaviors and restricted interests.[5] In addition to presenting with these core deficits, many individuals with ASD also suffer from comorbid disorders, including language disorders, behavioral problems, attention-deficit/hyperactivity disorder, depression, anxiety, and other psychiatric conditions.[7,8] This wide-ranging inclusion of comorbid features within a disorder that is described as a spectrum highlights the salient need for educators to consider each student's unique strengths and difficulties. Therefore, educating students diagnosed with ASD can be a complex undertaking that requires special training.

EDUCATIONAL PROGRAMS

The Autism Society of America (ASA) defines quality of life as "basic human rights that allow people to interact with one another and the world in their own terms."[9] One example of a quality-of-life indicator cited on the ASA Web site is academic success that is defined as "the opportunity to participate in school to one's fullest capability and learn in an environment that enables success."[9]

Some students with autism may access educational services and treatment in a general education setting whereas other may require special education services in a more restrictive setting. This is dependent on the level of supports a student needs to access curriculum. In 2014, data from the Centers for Disease Control and Prevention indicated that approximately 22% of 8-year-old children having a clinical ASD diagnosis also have an intellectual disability.[10] These data suggest that 78% may be academically capable. Based on this, Barnard-Brak and Reschly state, "academically capable students with no behavioral health needs and limited externalizing behavior concerns may not require services or an educational diagnosis to do well in school."[11] In 2015, the US Department of Education (DOE) estimated that approximately 40% of students with ASD were participating in the general education setting for at least 80% of the school day.[12] Kim and colleagues[13] concluded that children with ASD, including those with average or above-average IQ and achievement scores were more likely to move from general education or inclusion classrooms to full-time special education classrooms from ages 9 years to 18 years compared with those with non-ASD diagnoses.

Throughout the United States, there are a multitude of education programs available to individuals diagnosed with ASD. These programs include the general education setting, special education services within the general education setting, special education services within a separate special education setting, and intensive in-home teaching. All programs vary in implementation and outcomes and have advantages and disadvantages depending on the needs of the student. To identify an educational environment that can effectively teach a child with autism, Sundberg and Partington,[14] recommend that, "When considering options it is important to remember that there are several outcomes desired for any educational program. The most important outcome is that the child acquires skills that are both immediately useful to him and allow him to learn additional skills without highly trained staff and individualized instruction. Ideally, the child should acquire skills that enable him to learn from what he sees and hears every day, while interacting with a variety of individuals (eg, aunts, uncles, neighbors, peers). In order to meet these goals it is essential to identify an educational environment that can effectively teach the child."[14]

RESEARCH ON EVIDENCE-BASED PRACTICES

In 2001 The National Research Council (NRC) published a book entitled, *Educating Children with Autism* toward its mission "to improve government decision making and public policy, increase public education and understanding, and promote the acquisition and dissemination of knowledge in matters involving science, engineering, technology, and health."[15] The NRC book provides a summary of recommendations for children with autism from birth to age 8 years, across 7 areas, 2 of which are goals for educational services and characteristics of effective interventions:[16]

- Goals for educational services
  - Objective: observable, measureable behavior and skills
- Characteristics of effective interventions
  - Educational services; immediate, adapted, intensive, individually located
  - Sufficient individualized attention
  - Ongoing measurement of educational objectives
  - Specialized instruction with typically developing children
  - Six kinds of interventions should have priority

The identified 6 kinds of interventions that should have priority include functional, spontaneous communication; social instruction; teaching play skills; cognitive development; problem behavior; and functional academic skills. Furthermore, the NRC recommends that the content of curriculum for children with ASDs should be based on sound research[17] and that educational services should be a minimum of 25 hours per week, 12 months a year.[16]

In 2015, the National Autism Center (NAC) identified 14 evidence-based practices (EBPs) for children and youth with ASD in its National Standards Project, a project that sought to provide educators and others with the most current information on effective treatment of individuals with ASD.[18] The NAC mission is to "provide leadership and comprehensive evidence-based resources to families, practitioners, and policymakers, to programs and organizations, and to the national community."[18] The 14 treatments are behavioral interventions, cognitive behavioral interventions package, comprehensive behavioral treatment of young children, language training (production), modeling, naturalistic teaching strategies, parent training package, peer training package, pivotal response treatment, schedules, scripting, self-management, social skills package, and story-based intervention.[18]

From 2007 to 2014, the Office of Special Education Programs in the DOE funded the National Professional Development Center on Autism Spectrum Disorder (NPDC).[19] The goal was to advance the use of EBPs for individuals with ASD from birth to 22 years of age.[19] In 2015, the NPDC identified 27 EBPs as effective interventions when implemented with fidelity (**Table 1**). The EBPs identified by both the NAC and NPDC overlap and most fit in to the 6 priority intervention areas outlined in the NRC recommendations.

It is important for educators to understand the limitations of relying solely on EBPs,[38,39] including that what is meant by evidence-based may vary and that interventions not labeled as evidence-based might still be effective. Lubas and colleagues[8] point out that just because a strategy is evidence based does not mean it is effective for every student with ASD. Also, the implementation of EBPs may not take into account the individuality of students with ASD because the focus of EBPs is centered on research. Lubas and colleagues[8] believe the current "skewed focus" of research in EBPs does not account for teacher expertise or student characteristics, 2 additional critical facets of educational programming for students with ASD.

CURRICULUM

A challenge faced by both general and special educators is aligning educational programs for students with ASD to curriculum standards. This is the case particularly when the standards are as rigorous as the Common Core State Standards (CCSS), which have been adopted by 41 states as well as the District of Columbia during the past 9 years.[40] The CCSS provide information for what students should know/be able to learn by the end of each grade so, by the time they graduate high school, they have the skills to succeed in college, a career, or an alternative educational setting.[40]

Students with ASD characteristically demonstrate weak executive function, difficulty interpreting nonverbal cues, difficulty with perspective taking, and problems seeing the big picture.[41] Because of this, an educator working with students on the spectrum should understand how their particular set of strengths, challenges, and deficits can affect their ability to interact with curriculum. For example, a student may have a prolific vocabulary but have trouble comprehending simple instructions or may have strengths in decoding but difficulty with reading comprehension.[41] Furthermore, students with ASD may struggle with standards that require cognitive flexibility, analytical thinking, and/or increased processing speed.[41,42] In addition to understanding these curricular challenges it is important for teachers to be aware that many students with ASD "do not ask questions or seek help from others."[41] Therefore, it is crucial for educators to adapt the curriculum, modify instructional materials, and have a working knowledge of EBPs.[38,39,43,44]

Research conducted by Hudson and colleagues[45] showed promise for 2 evidence-based, instructional practices that can be used during math instruction. These involved the use of graphic organizers and manipulatives with a simultaneous prompting procedure. In a study conducted by Knight and colleagues,[46] task analysis, another identified, EBP, whether scripted or unscripted, was found to be successful for acquisition of science content. Constable and colleagues[41] recommended that educators use EBPs, such as prompting, visual supports, social narratives and comic strip conversations, naturalistic interventions, and peer-mediated instruction, to support and improve learning in English language arts.

Table 1
Twenty-seven evidence-based practices identified by the National Professional Development Center on Autism Spectrum Disorder

Intervention	Definition/Description
Antecedent-based intervention	A behavior change strategy that manipulates contingency-independent antecedent stimuli (motivating operations)[20]
Cognitive behavioral intervention	Teaches learners to examine their own thoughts and emotions, recognize when negative thoughts and emotions are escalating in intensity, and then use strategies to change their thinking and behavior.[21]
Differential reinforcement	A procedure for decreasing problem behavior in which reinforcement is contingent on the absence of the problem behavior during or at specific times[20]
Discrete trial training	An approach in which the instructor delivers 1 or multiple discriminative stimuli and, contingent on the appropriateness of the participant response, provides reinforcement or implements individualized prompting strategies[22]
Exercise	Can be used to improve the physical fitness of learners with ASD. In addition, exercise can be used to increase desired behaviors (time on task, correct responding) and decrease inappropriate behaviors (aggression, self-injury).[23]
Extinction	The discontinuation of a reinforcement of a previously reinforced behavior (ie, response no longer produces reinforcement); the primary effect is a decrease in the frequency of the behavior until it reaches a prereinforced level or ultimately ceases to occur.[20]
Functional behavior assessment	A systematic method of assessment for obtaining information about the purposes (functions) a problem behavior serves for a person; results are used to guide the design of an intervention for decreasing the problem behavior and increasing appropriate behavior[20]
Functional communication training	An antecedent intervention in which an appropriate communicative behavior is taught as a replacement behavior for problem behavior usually evoked by an establishing operation; involves differential reinforcement of alternative behavior[20]
Modeling	Demonstrating the desired behavior[24]
Naturalistic interventions	Incorporating instruction for individuals with disabilities into less structured activities[24]
Parent-implemented interventions	Practitioners collaborating with, training, and coaching parents to implement EBPs with their children throughout daily routines and activitie.[25]
Peer-mediated instruction and intervention	Systematically teaching peers without disabilities ways of engaging learners with ASD in positive and meaningful social interactions[26]
Picture exchange communication system	An alternative/augmentative communication system that was developed to teach functional communication to children with limited speech. The approach is unique in that it teaches children to initiate communicative interactions within a social framework.[27]
Pivotal response training	A naturalistic intervention that focuses on motivation, responsivity to multiple cues, self-management, and social initiations[28,29]
Prompting	Additional stimuli that increase the probability that a discriminative stimulus will occasion the desired response[24]

(continued on next page)

Table 1
(continued)

Intervention	Definition/Description
Reinforcement	Occurs when a stimulus change immediately follows a response and increases the future frequency of that type of behavior in similar conditions[20]
Response interruption/ redirection	A procedure in which the therapist physically intervenes as soon as the learner begins to emit a problem behavior to prevent completion of the targeted behavior[20]
Scripting	A visual or auditory cue that supports learners to initiate or sustain communication with others[30]
Self-management	The personal application of behavior change tactics that produces a desired change in behavior[20]
Social narratives	Describing social situations for learners by providing relevant cues, explanation of the feelings and thoughts of others, and descriptions of appropriate behavior expectations[26]
Social skills training	A therapeutic approach used to improve interpersonal relations[31]
Structured play groups	Small group activities with a defined area, activity, theme, and roles with typically developing peers and an adult scaffolding as needed to support the learner with ASD's performance[32]
Task analysis	Breaking a complex skill or series of behaviors into smaller, teachable units; also refers to the results of this process[20]
Technology-aided instruction and intervention	Refers to instruction or intervention in which technology is the central feature supporting the acquisition of a goal for the learner[33]
Time delay	A fading format used when prompting. Rather than presenting the prompt immediately, the teacher waits, thus allowing the student to respond before prompting.[24]
Video modeling	Involves a child watching a video of an adult, peer, or him/herself performing a target behavior and in turn displaying the behavior[34,35]
Visual supports	Can be in the form of objects, pictures, line drawings, or words[36] that are used to prompt and remind students to organize work and materials and/or engage in appropriate behavior or activities[37]

Data from The National Professional Development Center on Autism Spectrum Disorder. 2019. Available at https://autismpdc.fpg.unc.edu/evidence-based-practices. Accessed July 16, 2019.

Denning and Moody's[42] research suggests that students with ASD matriculated in the general education setting may benefit from support provided through the principles of Universal Design for Learning (UDL). The core features of UDL include multiple means of representation, action and expression, and engagement.[47] Denning and Moody[42] outlined several strategies that, when implemented within a UDL framework in an inclusive setting, yielded successful instructional outcomes for students with ASD. Some of the strategies included in their work are use of schedules, video modeling, interest-based lessons, visual supports, explicit instructions, modeling, and guided practice.[42]

AUTISM IN THE CLASSROOM

Children and youth with autism respond well to structure and thrive in classroom environments that are highly predictable.[36,48] Additionally, they may lack motivation, have difficulty engaging and filtering unnecessary information, habe trouble successfully completing work, demonstrate cognitive rigidity, and struggle with executive functioning.[42] TEACCH, formerly referred to as Treatment and Education of Autistic and Communication related handicapped CHildren, was cofounded in 1972 by Eric Schopler and colleagues, a pioneer in the field of autism education.[49] TEACCH is an evidence-based service that conducts research, trains professionals and families, and provides programming for individuals with ASD of all ages and abilities.[49,50] TEACCH has become a model for programs across the country and around the world. TEACCH emphasizes the importance of structured teaching by using schedules, visual structure, physical organization, and work systems.[50] The elements of structured teaching are intended to give the student a set of clear and consistent expectations in an orderly and predictable environment. Structured teaching also consists of highly individualized programming with the end goal of increasing an individual's independent functioning.[49,50]

Research indicates that individuals with ASD have strengths in visual processing[51] and are stronger visual learners than their typically developing peers,[49] making the use of visual supports vital to success in the classroom. One type of visual support that should be available to all students with autism is schedules. Sarahan and Copas state, "visual schedules and predictable routines help take the chaos out of the learning environment."[52] Furthermore, they assist with understanding and retaining verbal and sequenced information.[48,52] Schedules are visual cues to organizing tasks in temporal order (**Figs. 1** and **2**). When developing a schedule, teachers should consider each individual student's learning characteristics so the schedule is individualized and meaningful to the student. Therefore, considerations, such as form, cue to initiate use, location and portability, length, and method to manage, all must be taken in to account for each student. An effective schedule focuses on the development of independent skills (**Fig. 3**).[36,48] It organizes time, helps a student shift attention, and promotes tolerance and flexibility when the environment is less predictable.[36]

In addition to visual schedules, visual structure in the classroom is also vitally important. Young people with autism may experience confusion and/or distress when they are expected to process and follow verbal directions.[49] Research[53] indicates that children with ASD may present with a range of language delays in both expressive and receptive language and that young children with ASD have core deficits in joint attention and shared affect. Curiel and Sainato further assert that these delays could include "very limited speech, lack of response to social interactions, and deficits in understanding gestures."[54] The use of visual structure in the classroom can provide students with a strategy for approaching tasks differently and help draw attention to relevant information.[36,48] Visual structure involves the use of space and materials in a manner that helps limit the focus of attention (**Figs. 4** and **5**). Another is the use of visual presentations of information (**Figs. 6** and **7**). The use of written or picture instructions (**Fig. 8**), models, or cutout jigs provides students with a systematic strategy for work completion. Visual instructions help putting separate parts of the task together in the correct sequence (**Figs. 9** and **10**). The use of visual clarity emphasizes where to look (**Fig. 11**). Examples include highlighting information, indicating sequence, clarifying placement, and displaying clear indication of how/when a task is finished.

Another key component of structured teaching is physical organization.[49] This involves the arrangement of materials and the physical space. It is important for a classroom to have clearly defined areas so students can understand where they are supposed to be and what is expected of them in each area of the classroom. Careful considerations to the physical space can help control distractions and focus a student's attention. For example, furniture or partitions can be used to define boundaries

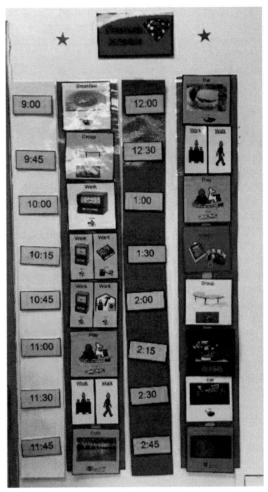

Fig. 1. This is a classroom schedule using photos, picture symbols, and words so that non-readers and readers know which activity occurs during each interval of the school day. (*Courtesy of* The Forbush School at Hunt Valley, Part of the Sheppard Pratt Health System, Towson, MD.)

and create smaller areas in a larger classroom (**Fig. 12**). Book shelves can be used to create a barrier between a leisure and instructional space. In addition to the physical layout and organization, environmental sensory stimuli should be considered. Students with autism display sensory sensitivities to environmental stimuli that affect their attention and engagement in classroom learning activities.[54] Sarahan and Copas[52] point out that careful consideration of lighting, sensory stimulation, classroom and play arrangements, and group structure is necessary. Kinneal and colleagues[55] concluded that there can be a positive effect on students' attention in the classroom when classroom walls are constructed with material that absorbs sound. Students who are sensitive to fluorescent lighting in the classroom may be less disturbed or distracted when magnetic, fabric panels are hung over the lights (**Fig. 13**). The panels help filter the light and reduce the flickering and glare typically produced by fluorescent lighting that can be bothersome and upsetting to some individuals with ASD.

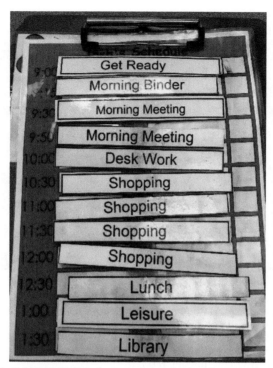

Fig. 2. This is an individual schedule for a student who is able to read. It identifies what is happening and when during the school day. It is on a clipboard so that it can be either stationary or portable. (*Courtesy of* The Forbush School at Hunt Valley, Part of the Sheppard Pratt Health System, Towson, MD.)

The final component of structured teaching is work systems. Work systems provide students with a systematic way to approach assignments.[56] The space is organized visually so that students can independently practice previously acquired skills. An effective work system answers 4 questions: What work? How much work? When am I finished? and What is next?[49,57] Furthermore, work systems are designed to enable generalization of skills to other environments. Teachers are advised to consider form, organization, and sequence; how progress is tracked by the student; and how the transition after task completion is indicated when creating work systems for their students. **Fig. 14** shows a color-coded work system. This work system was designed for 5 different students to complete 4 different tasks each. During work time, each student is provided with a corresponding visual schedule that indicates the color and 4 tasks they are assigned to complete. In their study, Park and Kim[56] found that the work systems could contribute to reducing disruptive behaviors and promoting independent, sustained engagement for participants. When Hume and colleagues[57] used work systems as an intervention for first-grade students, less adult assistance was needed and students achieved more accurate object/photo classification and sight word recognition.

When incorporating any element of structured teaching, TEACCH recommends that educators integrate students' strengths and interests. Denning and Moody[42] suggest that teachers spend time learning each student's special interests and use them for classroom activities and readings in an effort to enhance and maintain engagement in classroom assignments. Mancil and Pearl[58] believe that "Embedding restricted

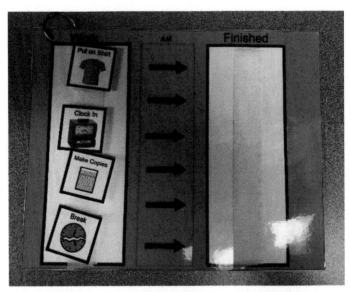

Fig. 3. This schedule is for a student who is learning to complete multiple steps to a task with greater independence. As students complete each step, they move the picture symbol to the finished side. The use of a visual schedule allows a teacher to provide less intrusive prompting as a student as moves through the tasks. The break picture at the end is the reinforcer for work completion. (*Courtesy of* The Forbush School at Hunt Valley, Part of the Sheppard Pratt Health System, Towson, MD.)

interests into activities as motivators can help children with ASD stay engaged during academic activities."[58] The work area shown in **Fig. 15** was designed specifically for a student who engages in out-of-seat behavior in an attempt to hide from teachers. The sheet tied around the legs of the desk provides the student with an opportunity to "hide" while remaining in location. This small modification to the work area increased motivation to stay in the work area and be more consistently available for instruction. Lanou and colleagues state, "Educators can embrace students' unique humor, idiosyncratic interests, and seemingly 'nonfunctional' behaviors to motivate them in meeting challenging social and academic expectations while also increasing their confidence and independence."[51]

One case study, described in Lanou, Hough, and Powell's research as the "Iceberg Cue," capitalized on Jimmy's interest in the RMS Titanic to develop his awareness of personal space. Teachers and peers would use the phrase "iceberg right ahead" when Jimmy would begin to encroach on someone's personal space. This intervention resulted in a significant decrease in Jimmy entering his peers' personal space.[51] Mancil and Pearl[58] shared that by tapping into students' interests, teachers at the elementary, middle, and high school levels experienced an increase in sustained engagement in academic instruction and marked improvements in reading, history, science, and math for their students with ASD. Preece and Howley[59] discovered that understanding the individuality of each student with ASD and appealing to each student's interests is key to helping students with high rates of absenteeism reengage in formal education.

When incorporating students' interests into academic instruction, factors to be considered include the appropriateness of the interest as it relates to the academic outcome, whether and how the restricted interest may interfere with peer

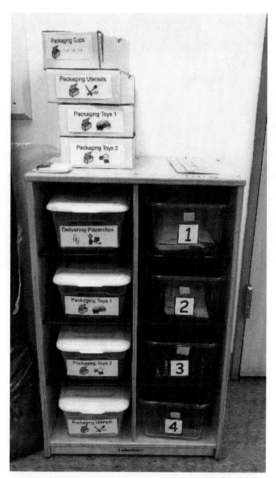

Fig. 4. This is a student's work system. The bins on the left are labeled with picture symbols and there is a corresponding set of index cards with identical picture symbols on top of the shelf. During work, the student is provided with a set of index cards indicating which work she needs to be complete. The bins on the right are labeled with yellow numbers 1 to 4. There is a corresponding visual schedule located above the bins that the student uses to move through her work. Through color coding and matching numbers, the student is able to complete all the required tasks during work with independence. (*Courtesy of* The Forbush School at Hunt Valley, Part of the Sheppard Pratt Health System, Towson, MD.)

relationships, and the age appropriateness of the interest.[58] Atwood[60] (2007) suggests that a child's or youth's restrictive interests may serve

- To overcome anxiety
- To provide pleasure
- To provide relaxation
- To ensure greater predictability and certainty in life
- To help understand the physical world
- To create an alternative world
- To create a sense of identity
- To occupy time, facilitate conversation, and indicate intellectual ability[60]

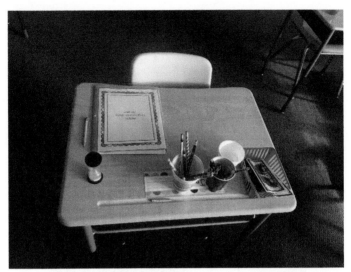

Fig. 5. The cups and bins on this student's desk are used to organize and store materials. The cups store pencils, which this student likes to collect. The plastic bin holds the "money" the student earns as a reward for expected behavior. The hourglass timer is used as needed so the student is able to see how much time she has for breaks. (*Courtesy of* The Forbush School at Hunt Valley, Part of the Sheppard Pratt Health System, Towson, MD.)

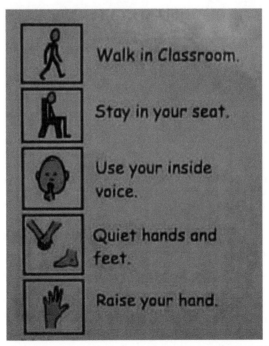

Fig. 6. This is a visual presentation of the rules students are expected to follow while in class. (*Courtesy of* The Forbush School at Hunt Valley, Part of the Sheppard Pratt Health System, Towson, MD.)

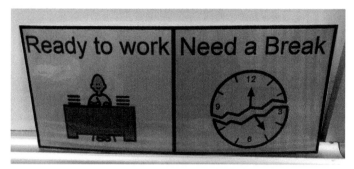

Fig. 7. This visual aid is used by students and/or staff. Students are able to indicate their readiness for learning and staff are able to ask students if they are ready to work or if they need a break. (*Courtesy of* The Forbush School at Hunt Valley, Part of the Sheppard Pratt Health System, Towson, MD.)

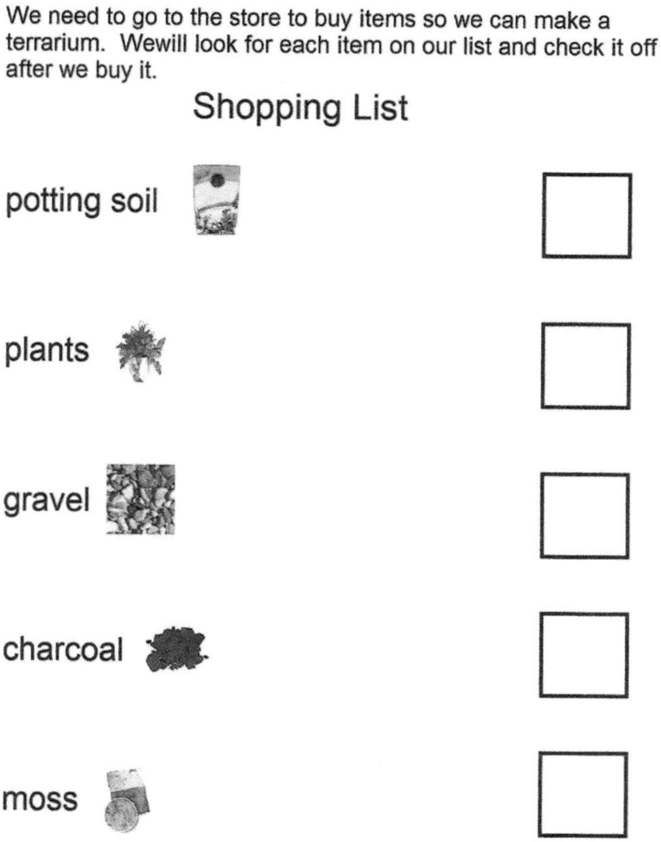

We need to go to the store to buy items so we can make a terrarium. We will look for each item on our list and check it off after we buy it.

Shopping List

potting soil

plants

gravel

charcoal

moss

Fig. 8. This shopping list uses both words and pictures so that both readers and nonreaders can refer to it while shopping. As they find each item at the store, they can put a check or mark the box to indicate completion of the task. (*Courtesy of* The Forbush School at Hunt Valley, Part of the Sheppard Pratt Health System, Towson, MD.)

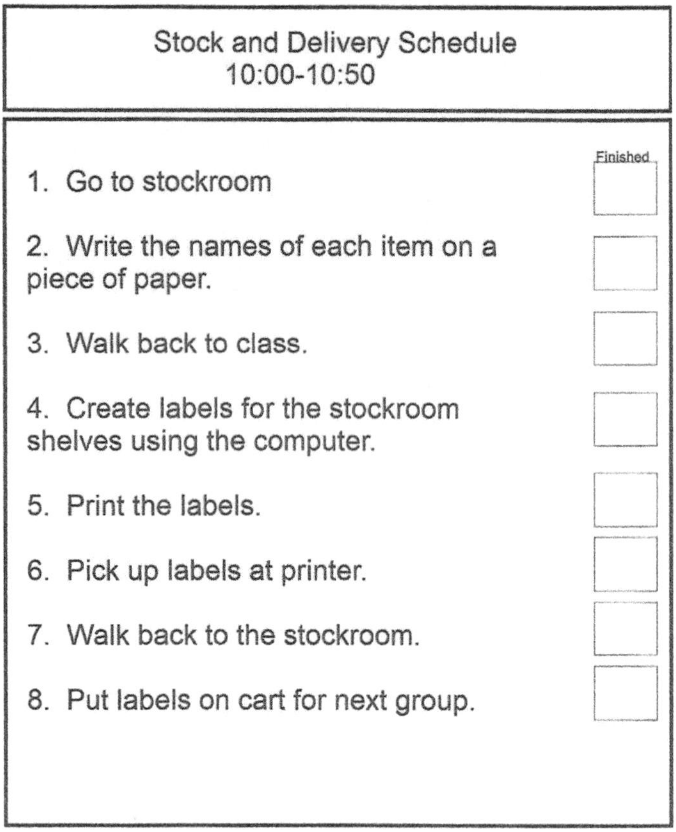

```
┌─────────────────────────────────────────────────┐
│              Stock and Delivery Schedule          │
│                   10:00-10:50                     │
└─────────────────────────────────────────────────┘
```

	Finished
1. Go to stockroom	☐
2. Write the names of each item on a piece of paper.	☐
3. Walk back to class.	☐
4. Create labels for the stockroom shelves using the computer.	☐
5. Print the labels.	☐
6. Pick up labels at printer.	☐
7. Walk back to the stockroom.	☐
8. Put labels on cart for next group.	☐

Fig. 9. This is a set of written instructions for a student to follow to complete a school-based job. As the student completes each step, a checkmark is placed in the box. (*Courtesy of* The Forbush School at Hunt Valley, Part of the Sheppard Pratt Health System, Towson, MD.)

When restricted interested cannot be part of instruction, research[58] suggests that teachers consider following the Premack principle and using the individual's restricted interest as a reinforcer.

There are advantages and disadvantages to implementing components of TEACCH in the classroom and its effects may vary across domains. TEACCH provides a range of approaches rather than there being a universal curriculum that every student should try to fit into.[61] Results from a study conducted by Boyd and colleagues[62] yielded an interesting finding: children who received lower baseline Mullen scale scores made greater gains than their higher scoring peers when enrolled in TEACCH classrooms. The Mullen Scales of Early Learning are an assessment tool that provides a quick, reliable measure of motor development and cognitive ability for infants through age 68 months. This may suggest "that some of the environmental and behavioral supports used in TEACCH are more beneficial to children with greater cognitive impairments."[62] Furthermore, a study conducted by Park and Kim[56] suggests that TEACCH-structured teaching improved independent engagement and reduced disruptive behavior in 3 young adults with severe autism. Virues-Ortega and colleagues[63] conducted a meta-anfalysis and determined that TEACCH methods yielded greater gains in the areas of social and maladaptive behaviors versus communication,

---

Friday Library Schedule

Finished

1. Walk to the library.

2. Get the blue cart.

3. Walk to each classroom to collect library books.
   Say, "Do you have any library books?

4. Put returned library books in to the correct classroom bin by matching numbers.

5. Bring the cart back to the library.

6. Check the books in.

7. Sort the books by subject/topic/theme.

8. Put the books back on the shelves in the correct area.

Fig. 10. This is a set of written instructions for a student to follow to complete a school-based job. As the student completes each step, a checkmark is placed in the box. (*Courtesy of* The Forbush School at Hunt Valley, Part of the Sheppard Pratt Health System, Towson, MD.)

motor, perceptual, or adaptive skills. These varying outcomes help to highlight how critical it is for educators to individualize instruction for students with ASD.

APPLIED BEHAVIOR ANALYSIS

Applied behavior analysis (ABA) is one of the most empirically validated forms of treatment of educating individuals with ASD.[64] ABA is an EBP that distinguishes itself from experimental analysis of behavior "by its focus on solving socially important problems in socially important settings."[65] ABA is widely used to educate children and youth with ASD because of its emphasis on social impact and its reliance on making data-based decisions. Cooper and colleagues define ABA as "the scientific approach for discovering environmental variables that reliably influence socially significant behavior and for developing a technology of behavior change that takes practical advantage of those discoveries."[20(p3)]

The application of ABA interventions for children and youth with autism dates back to the 1960s. Within the field of autism, Dr Ole Ivar Løvaas was a strong and early proponent of the use of discrete trial training, an approach in which the instructor delivers

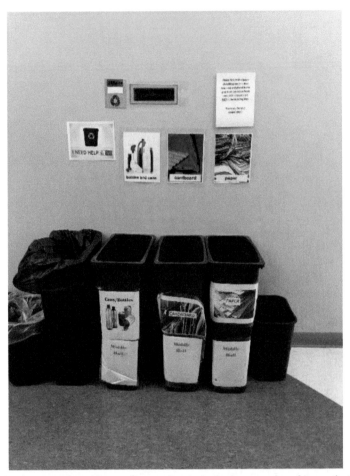

Fig. 11. Visuals are used at this recycling station to indicate examples of items that are recyclable and to clarify placement of items that are recycled. (*Courtesy of* The Forbush School at Hunt Valley, Part of the Sheppard Pratt Health System, Towson, MD.)

1 or multiple discriminative stimuli and, contingent on the appropriateness of the participant's response, provides reinforcement or implements individualized prompting strategies.[22] Ivar Lovaas and his colleagues were able to demonstrate that, with an effective intervention, children with ASD could make social and intellectual gains.[64] Many of the NPDC-identified EBPs[18] are "foundational applied behavior analysis techniques,"[66] These include antecedent-based intervention, differential reinforcement, extinction, functional communication training, pivotal response training, prompting, reinforcement, task analysis (**Fig. 16**), and time delay.[20,35,46,65]

The gap between research and practice can be a limitation to the use of ABA in school settings.[65] Some interventions rooted in ABA can be difficult to implement in a classroom setting whereas others can be simpler for teachers to implement (eg, pivotal response training).[29] An added limitation may be the lack of teacher preparedness and training in the principles of ABA. Often, ABA programs are developed and overseen by a Board Certified Behavior Analyst (BCBA). BCBAs receive extensive and systematized education, training, and supervision as they pursue their license.[67]

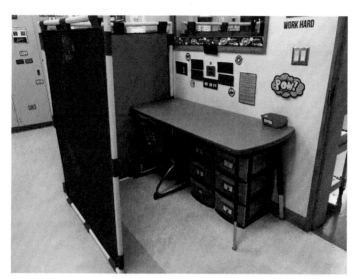

Fig. 12. Partitions are used to create a student's work space in a large classroom. (*Courtesy of* The Forbush School at Hunt Valley, Part of the Sheppard Pratt Health System, Towson, MD.)

The training a BCBA receives is not commensurate with that of a teacher, particularly as it relates to programming for students with ASD. Despite these limitations, there still is a significant amount of evidence to support that procedures based on the principles of ABA are representative of effective EBPs for individuals on the spectrum.[65,67]

BEHAVIOR CHANGE IN THE CLASSROOM

Both general and special educators may experience a wide range of behaviors from the ASD students in their classrooms. Some students with autism may engage in severe, dangerous, and challenging behaviors that can be disruptive to the classroom and contribute to academic failure.[68] Research suggests that 10% to 15% of individuals with an intellectual disability exhibit challenging behaviors, including aggression, self-injurious behavior, and destructive behavior.[69,70] Other students

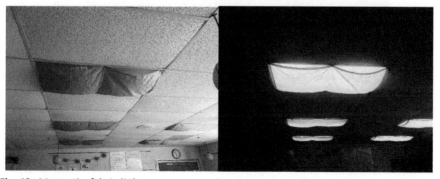

Fig. 13. Magnetic, fabric light covers are used to decrease sensitivity to fluorescent lights in a classroom. (*Courtesy of* The Forbush School at Hunt Valley, Part of the Sheppard Pratt Health System, Towson, MD.)

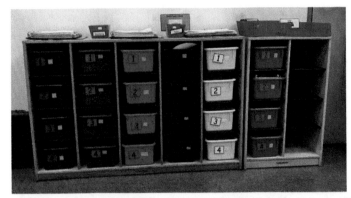

Fig. 14. This is a color-coded work system. This work system is designed for 5 different students to complete 4 different tasks each by using visual schedules that correspond to the numbers and color-coding on the bins. (*Courtesy of* The Forbush School at Hunt Valley, Part of the Sheppard Pratt Health System, Towson, MD.)

may engage in behaviors, such as repetitive movements or scripting, that do not pose a safety risk but are disruptive. Schopler and colleagues[71] contend that students tend to make steady academic progress when their idiosyncratic behaviors are accepted by their teachers and, therefore, teachers should focus only on those behaviors that interfere with learning. For example, when a behavior like finger tapping is ignored and accepted by teachers, a student with ASD may flourish academically.[71]

It is thus important for educators to be prepared for their students with autism to exhibit disruptive and challenging behaviors. When teachers are not prepared, these behaviors pose risks for students of academic failure, poor social supports, restrictive

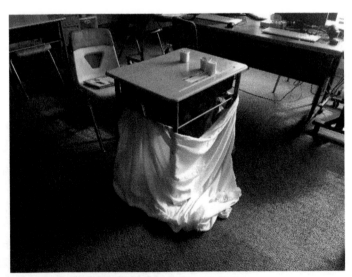

Fig. 15. The sheet tied around the legs of this student's desk allows her to "hide" when she is feeling overwhelmed. "Hiding" is a replacement behavior she is offered to do instead of leaving her seat or eloping from the classroom. (*Courtesy of* The Forbush School at Hunt Valley, Part of the Sheppard Pratt Health System, Towson, MD.)

Task/Skill: Objective:				SD: Mastery Criteria: 3 consecutive independent responses				Chaining Procedure: TT F B Instructions:			
Date: Staff Initials: Step:											
1											
2											
3											

Fig. 16. Prompt hierarchy: B, backward chaining; F, forward chaining; FP, full physical prompt; GP, gestural prompt: I, independent; MP, model prompt; PP, partial physical prompt; TT, total task chaining. (*Courtesy of* The Forbush School at Hunt Valley, Part of the Sheppard Pratt Health System, Towson, MD.)

behavioral techniques, medications possibly with significant side effects, and/or disproportionate rates of suspension.[68] Preparing teachers with the tools and skills required to effectively teach students with autism can be particularly challenging because students with ASD are a heterogeneous group.[72] Woolfson[73] indicates that teachers often convey feelings of anxiety regarding teacher preparedness. Teacher training needs to focus on EBPs to meet the academic, social, and language needs of students with autism. Denning and Moody state, "Today's classrooms are increasingly diverse and teachers need to proactively set-up the environment and instructional methods in ways that support all learners."[42] Therefore, it is imperative for all educators to be equipped to teach students with autism, including having an understanding of the components of a classroom that make it more conducive to students with autism. Effective teacher preparation programs should be ever evolving so that teachers stay motivated. Busby and colleagues state,

If teachers have superior training, preparation and experiences, and are provided the tools to facilitate success, they will begin to feel more confident in their abilities to teach children with autism and other disabilities. Teachers will feel empowered and the challenges that they face will become less daunting.[74]

POSTSECONDARY

Many individuals with ASD struggle with change.[75,76] According to Marsh and colleagues[77] starting school is a major event that can be particularly challenging for individuals with ASD. For youth with autism who are transitioning to their postsecondary years, this transition can be exacerbated by several other factors. There is research to support that the life beyond high school can be bleak.[76] According to Shattuck and colleagues,[78] 35% of young adults (ages 19–23) with autism have not had a job or received postgraduate education after leaving high school and they were most as risk for being fully detached from all postsecondary opportunities.

When students exit school with a high school diploma or alternative certificate, they are no longer entitled to the same educational services and funding they were entitled to under the Individuals with Disabilities Education Act (IDEA) during their kindergarten through 12th-grade years. This results in challenges for families as the responsibility to continue to provide support to their child during this transition lies with them.[76] Additionally, according to Lounds and colleagues,[79] this transition period can cause increased anxiety for mothers of children with ASD, and research[76] has concluded that when there is more negativity than positivity in the family home, this had an impact on the occurrence of problem behaviors for youth with ASD. For individuals with ASD, as they continue to mature and navigate this postsecondary transition, they continue to face challenges similar to those they faced when they were enrolled in school. Just because the calendar changed does not mean a student changed or that the supports they were provided the day or month before are no longer needed.

Research by White and colleagues[80] emphasizes the importance of planning for a transition from high school to postsecondary opportunities. In 1997, IDEA was reauthorized and mandated that individualized education plans include transition planning to begin at age 14 and include a transition services component at age 16.[81–83] Therefore, it is the responsibility of school professionals to help ensure that students who have a disability and receive special education services be part of transition planning that begins early in their high school years. In order for this transition to be optimal, all aspects of the transition plan should be participant driven to the greatest extent possible.[84] Flexibility and individualization in incorporating students' strengths and interests is vital to meeting their unique needs.[83]

Research on postsecondary outcomes indicates that adaptive functioning, IQ, and psychiatric comorbidity are significant predictors of postsecondary success for individuals with ASD.[85] Furthermore, a study conducted by Zukerman and colleagues found that "lower adaptive functioning was associated with the severity of social anxiety and obsessive compulsive symptoms in ASD participants."[85] These findings stress the importance of continued access to instruction in independent living skills and social emotional behavior beyond the high school.

SUMMARY

The passage of laws pertaining to individuals with disabilities has opened the door for greater opportunity for children and youth diagnosed with ASDs to receive the specialized and individualized educational services that yield successful outcomes. It is evident that there is still no 1 best practice for educating individuals with autism due to the spectrum and variety of symptoms experienced by those with ASD and the need for highly individualized programming. Although there is a wide breadth of research on educating children and youth with autism, more is necessary for educators and the pubic to gain a greater understanding of the wide range of outcomes that exist. There is particular need for additional studies beyond school-aged children because educating a person with ASD does not stop at high school graduation; it is a lifelong pursuit.

REFERENCES

1. Melvin DH. The desegregation of children with disabilities. DePaul Law Review 1995;44(2):590–671.
2. Yell ML, Rogers D, Lodge-Rogers E. The legal history of special education: what a long strange trip it's been! Remedial Spec Educ 1998;19:219–28.
3. Forte JL. History of special education: important landmark cases. Connecticut Lawyer. p. 26–9. Available at: http://www.fortelawgroup.com/history-special-education-important-landmark-cases/. Accessed February 4, 2020.

4. Grandin T. Thinking in pictures: my life with autism. New York: Vintage Books; 2006 (Original work published in 1995).

5. American Psychiatric Association. Diagnostic and statistical manual of mental disorders. 5th edition. Washington, DC: American Psychiatric Association; 2013.

6. Park HR, Lee JM, Moon HE, et al. A short review on the current understanding of autism spectrum disorders. Exp Neurobiol 2016;25(1):1–13.

7. Steensel FJA, Bogels SM, de Bruin EI. Psychiatric comorbidity in children with autism spectrum disorders: a comparison with children with ADHD. J Child Fam Stud 2013;22(3):368–76.

8. Lubas M, Mitchell J, De Leo G. Evidence-based practice for teachers of children with autism: a dynamic approach. Intervention in School and Clinic; 2015. p. 1–6. Available at: https://augusta.pure.elsevier.com/en/publications/evidence-based-practice-for-teachers-of-children-with-autism-a-dy. Accessed February 4, 2020.

9. Autism Society - quality of life outcomes. 2019. Available at: https://www.autism-society.org/. Accessed July 6, 2019.

10. Baio J, Wiggins L, Christensen DL, et al. Prevalence of autism spectrum disorder among children aged 8 years — autism and developmental disabilities monitoring network, 11 sites, United States, 2014. MMWR Surveill Summ 2018; 67(6):1–23.

11. Barnard-Brak L. Educational versus clinical diagnoses of autism spectrum disorder: updated and expanded findings. School Psychology Review 2019;48(2): 185–9.

12. National Center for Education Statistics. Fast facts students with disabilities, inclusion of. 2019. Available at: https://nces.ed.gov/fastfacts/display.asp?id=59. Accessed August 14, 2019.

13. Kim SH, Bal VH, Lord C. Longitudinal follow-up of academic achievement in children with autism from 2 to 18. J Child Psychol Psychiatry 2018;59(3):258–67.

14. Sundberg ML, Partington JW. Teaching language to children with autism and other developmental disabilities. Concord (CA): AVB Press; 1998.

15. The national Academies of science engineering medicine. 2019. Available at: http://www.nationalacademies.org/nasem. Accessed July 16, 2019.

16. Lord C, McGee JP. Educating children with autism. Washington, DC: National Academy Press; 2001.

17. Tincani M, Bloomfield Cucchiarra M, Thurman SK, et al. Evaluating NRC's recommendations for educating children with autism a decade later. Child Youth Care Forum 2014;43:315–37.

18. National autism center at may Institute. 2019. Available at: https://www.nationalautismcenter.org. Accessed July 16, 2019.

19. The national professional development center on autism spectrum disorder. 2019. Available at: https://autismpdc.fpg.unc.edu/evidence-based-practices. Accessed July 16, 2019.

20. Cooper JO, Heron TE, Heward WL. Applied behavior analysis. 2nd edition. Upper Saddle River (NJ): Pearson Education, Inc; 2007.

21. Mussey J, Dawkins T, AFIRM Team. Cognitive behavioral intervention. Chapel Hill (NC): National Professional Development Center on Autism Spectrum Disorder, FPG Child Development Center, University of North Carolina; 2017. Available at: http://afirm.fpg.unc.edu/cognitive-behavioral-intervention.

22. Dixon MR, Wiggins SH, Belisle J. The effectiveness of the peak relational training system and corresponding changes in the VB-MAPP for young adults with autism. J Appl Behav Anal 2018;51(2):321–34.

23. Griffin W, AFIRM Team. Exercise. Chapel Hill (NC): National Professional Development Center on Autism Spectrum Disorder, FPG Child Development Center, University of North Carolina; 2015. Available at: http://afirm.fpg.unc.edu/exercise.

24. Alberto PA, Troutman AC. Applied behavior analysis for teachers. 9th edition. Upper Saddle River (NJ): Pearson Education, Inc; 2013.

25. Amsbary J, AFIRM Team. Parent implemented interventions. Chapel Hill (NC): National Professional Development Center on Autism Spectrum Disorder, FPG Child Development Center, University of North Carolina; 2017. Available at: http://afirm.fpg.unc.edu/parent-implemented-interventions.

26. Sam A, AFIRM Team. Social narratives. Chapel Hill (NC): National Professional Development Center on Autism Spectrum Disorder, FPG Child Development Center, University of North Carolina; 2015. Available at: http://afirm.fpg.unc.edu/social-narratives.

27. Bondy A, Frost L. The picture exchange communication system. Behav Modif 2001;25(5):725–44.

28. Koegel RL, Bimbela A, Schreibman L. Collateral effects of parent training on family interactions. J Autism Dev Disord 1996;26(3):347–59.

29. Brock ME, Dueker SA, Barzak MA. Brief report: improving social outcomes for students with autism at recess through peer-mediated pivotal response training. J Autism Dev Disord 2018;48:2224–30.

30. Griffin W, AFIRM Team. Scripting. Chapel Hill (NC): National Professional Development Center on Autism Spectrum Disorder, FPG Child Development Center, University of North Carolina; 2017. Available at: http://afirm.fpg.unc.edu/scripting.

31. Kolakowsky-Hayner SA. Social skills training. In: Kreutzer JS, DeLuca J, Caplan B, editors. Encyclopedia of clinical neuropsychology. New York: Springer; 2011. p. 171–203.

32. Sam A, Kucharczyk S, Waters V, AFIRM Team. Structured play groups. Chapel Hill (NC): National Professional Development Center on Autism Spectrum Disorder, FPG Child Development Center, University of North Carolina; 2018. Available at: http://afirm.fpg.unc.edu/structured-play-groups.

33. Hedges S, AFIRM Team. Technology-aided instruction and intervention. Chapel Hill (NC): National Professional Development Center on Autism Spectrum Disorder, FPG Child Development Center, University of North Carolina; 2017. Available at: http://afirm.fpg.unc.edu/technology-aided-instruction-and-intervention.

34. Rex C, Charlop MH, Spector V. Using video modeling as an anti-bullying intervention for children with autism spectrum disorder. J Autism Dev Disord 2018;48:2701–13.

35. Halle S, Ninness C, Ninness SK, et al. Teaching social skills to students with autism: a video modeling social stories approach. Behav Social Issues 2016;25:42–63.

36. Cohen A, Demchak A. Use of visual supports to increase task independence in students with severe disabilities in inclusive educational settings. Educ Train Autism Dev Disabil 2018;53(1):84–99.

37. Callahan K, Shukla-Mehta S, Magee S, et al. ABA versus TEACCH: the case for defining and validating comprehensive treatment models in autism. J Autism Dev Disord 2010;40:74–88.

38. Myles BS, Grossman BG, Aspy R, et al. Planning a comprehensive program for students with autism spectrum disorders using evidence-based practices. Educ Train Austim Dev Disabil 2007;42(4):398–409.

39. Odom SL, Collet-Klingenberg L, Rogers SJ, et al. Evidence-based practices in interventions for children and youth with autism spectrum disorders. Prev Sch Fail 2010;54(4):275–82.

40. Common core state standards initiative preparing America's students for college & career – standards in Your state. Available at: http://www.corestandards.org/standards-in-your-state/. Accessed September 2, 2019.

41. Constable S, Grossi B, Moniz A, et al. Meeting the common core state standards for students with autism: the challenge for educators. Teach Exceptional Child 2013;45(3):6–13.

42. Denning CB, Moody AK. Supporting students with autism spectrum disorders in inclusive settings: rethinking instruction and design. Electronic Journal for Inclusive Education 2013;3(1):1–22.

43. Guldberg K. Evidence-based practice in autism educational research: can we bridge the research and practice gap. Oxford Rev Education 2017;43(2):149–61.

44. Smith RL. Evidence-based practices and students with autism spectrum disorders. Focus Autism Other Dev Disabil 2005;20(3):140–9.

45. Hudson ME, Rivera CJ, Grady MM. Research on mathematics instruction with students with significant cognitive disabilities: has anything changed? Res Pract Persons Severe Disabl 2018;43(1):38–53.

46. Knight VF, Collins B, Spriggs AD, et al. Scripted and unscripted science lessons for children with autism and intellectual disability. J Autism Dev Disord 2018;48:2542–57.

47. Jordan-Anstead ME. Teachers perceptions of barriers to universal design for learning. Walden dissertations and doctoral studies collection 2016. Available at: https://scholarworks.waldenu.edu/cgi/viewcontent.cgi?article=3002&context=dissertations Accessed February 4, 2020.

48. Rao SM, Gagie B. Learning through seeing and doing – visual supports for children with autism. Teach Exceptional Child 2006;38(6):26–33.

49. Mesibov GB, Shea V. Evidence-based practices and autism. Autism 2011;15(1):114–33.

50. D'Elia L, Valeri G, Sonnino F, et al. A longitudinal study of the TEACCH program in different settings: the potential benefits of low intensity intervention in preschool children with autism spectrum disorder. J Autism Dev Disord 2014;44:615–26.

51. Lanou A, Hough L, Powell E. Case studies on using strengths and interests to address the needs of students with autism spectrum disorders. Interv Sch Clin 2011;47(3):175–82.

52. Sarahan N, Copas R. Autism assets. Reclaiming Child Youth 2014;22(4):34–7.

53. Wetherby AM, Woods JJ. Early social interaction project for children with autism spectrum disorders beginning in the second year of life: a preliminary study. Topics in Early Childhood Special Education 2006;26(2):67–82.

54. Curiel ES, Sainato DM, Goldstein H. Matrix training of receptive language skills with a toddler with autism spectrum disorder: a case study. Education Treat Child 2016;39(1):95–109.

55. Kinnealey M, Pfeiffer B, Miller J, et al. Effect of classroom modification on attention and engagement of students with autism or dyspraxia. Am J Occup Ther 2012;66:511–9.

56. Park I, Kim Y. Effects of TEACCH structured teaching on independent work skills among individuals with severe disabilities. Educ Train Autism Dev Disabil 2018;53(4):343–52.

57. Hume K, Plavnick J, Odom SL. Promoting task acc1uracy and independence in students with autism across educational setting through the use of individual work systems. J Autism Dev Disord 2012;42:2084–99.

58. Mancil GR, Pearl CE. Restricted interests as motivators: improving academic engagement and outcomes of children on the autism spectrum. Teaching Exceptional Children Plus 2008;4(6):1–15.

59. Preece D, Howley M. An approach to supporting young people with autism spectrum disorder and high anxiety to re-engage with formal education – the impact on young people and their families. Int J Adolesc Youth 2018;23(4):468–81.

60. Atwood T. The complete guide to asperger's syndrome. Philadelphia: Jessica Kingley Publishers; 2007. p. 172–201.

61. Butler C. The effectiveness of the TEACCH approach in supporting the development of communication skills for learners with severe intellectual disabilities. Support Learn 2018;31(3):185–201.

62. Boyd B, Hume K, McBee T, et al. Comparative efficacy of LEAP, TEACCH and non-model-specific special education programs for preschoolers with autism spectrum disorders. J Autism Dev Disord 2014;44:366–80.

63. Virues-Ortega J, Julio FM, Pastor-Barriuso R. The TEACCH program for children and adults with autism: a meta-analysis of intervention studies. Clin Psychol Rev 2013;33(8):940–53.

64. Rosenwasser B, Axelrod S. The contributions of applied behavior analysis to the education of people with autism. Behav Modif 2001;25(5):671–7.

65. Slocum TA, Detrich R, Wilczynski SM, et al. The evidence-based practice of applied behavior analysis. Behav Analyst 2014;37:41–56.

66. Wong C, Odom SL, Hume KA, et al. Evidence-based practices for children, youth, and young adults with autism spectrum disorder: a comprehensive review. J Autism Dev Disord 2015;45:1951–66.

67. Blydenburg DM, Diller JW. Evaluating components of behavior-analytic training programs. Behav Anal Pract 2016;9:179–83.

68. Stevenson BS, Wood CL, Ianello AC. Effects of function-based crisis intervention on the severe challenging behavior of students with autism. Education Treat Child 2019;42(3):321–44.

69. Holden B, Gitlesen JP. A total population study of challenging behaviour in the county of Hedmark, Norway: prevalence, and risk markers. Res Dev Disabil 2006;27(4):456–65.

70. Emerson E, Kiernan C, Alborz AA, et al. The prevalence of challenging behaviors: a total population study. Res Dev Disabil 2001;22(1):77–93.

71. Schopler E, Mesibov G, Baker A. Evaluation of treatment for autistic children and their parents. J Am Acad Child Psychiatry 1982;21(3):262–7.

72. Morrier MJ, Hess KL, Heflin J. Teacher training for implementation of teaching strategies for students with autism spectrum disorders. Teach Educ Spec Educ 2011;34(2):119–32.

73. Woolfson L. Beyond formal assessment in inclusive classrooms: the complex relationship between teacher beliefs and teaching. Psychol Education Rev 2018;42(2):28–32.

74. Busby R, Ingram R, Bowron R, et al. Teaching elementary children with autism: addressing teacher challenges and preparation needs. Rural Educator 2012;33(2):27–34.

75. Hume K, Sreckovic M, Snyder K, et al. Smooth transitions helping students with autism spectrum disorder navigate the school day. Teach Exceptional Child 2014;47(1):1–11.

76. Smith L, Greenberg JS, Mailick MR. Adults with autism: outcomes, family effects, and the multi-family group psychoeducation model. Curr Psychiatry Rep 2012; 14(6):732–8.

77. Marsh A, Spagnol V, Grove R, et al. Transition to school for children with autism spectrum disorder: a systematic review. World J Psychiatry 2017;7(3):184–96.

78. Shattuck PT, Narendorf SC, Cooper B, et al. Postsecondary education and employment among youth with an autism spectrum disorder. Am Acad Pediatr 2012;129(6):1042–9.

79. Lounds J, Seltzer MM, Greenberg JS. Transition and change in adolescents and young adults with autism: longitudinal effects on maternal well-being. Am J Ment Retard 2007;112(6):401–17.

80. White SW, Elias R, Salinas CE, et al. Students with autism spectrum disorder in college: results from a preliminary mixed methods: needs analysis. Res Dev Disabil 2016;56:29–40.

81. Hasazi SB, DeStefano L, Furney KS. Implementing the IDEA transition mandates. In: Johnson DR, Emanuel EJ, editors. Issues influencing the future of transition programs and services in the United States: a collection of articles by leading researchers in secondary special education and transition services for students with disabilities. University of Minnesota: National Transition Network, Institute on Community Integration (UAP); 2000. p. 25–34.

82. Turnbull HR. Individuals with disabilities education act reauthorization: account and personal responsibility. Remedial Spec Education 2005;26(6):320–6.

83. T.E.C. Smith. IDEA 2004: another round in the reauthorization process. Remedial and Special Education 26(6):314–9.

84. White SW, Elias R, Capriola NN, et al. Development of a college transition and support program for students with autism spectrum disorder. J Autism Dev Disord 2017;47(10):3072–8.

85. Zukerman G, Yahav G, Ben-Itzchak EB. Increased psychiatric symptoms in university students with autism spectrum disorder are associated with reduced adaptive behavior. Psychiatry Res 2019;273:732–8.

The Transition to Adulthood for Young People with Autism Spectrum Disorder

Robert Wisner-Carlson, MD[a],*, Sara Uram, LCSW-C[b],
Thomas Flis, MS, BCBA, LBA, LCPC[c]

KEYWORDS

- Autism • ASD • Transition • Emerging adulthood • Social cognition
- Executive function • Adaptive function

KEY POINTS

- Transitions are inherently difficult for individuals with autism spectrum disorder (ASD), and outcomes in adulthood for individuals with ASD are suboptimal.
- Deficits in social cognition and executive function cause various problems as the expectations of early adulthood become more complex and supportive services fall off a cliff.
- All areas of adulthood are affected for individuals with ASD, including further education, employment, adaptive functioning, instrumental activities of daily living, social relations, sexuality, and more.
- Social skills training, employment interventions, college transition programs, and driver training technologies are examples of interventions, some of which are recommendable as best practices.
- Autism is not a rare disorder. With nearly 1.7% of 8-year-olds being identified by the Centers for Disease Control and Prevention as having ASD, it is incumbent on all psychiatrists—child, adolescent, and adult—to understand autism and the special needs and services this population requires to thrive throughout the life span.

INTRODUCTION

Life is filled with—and defined by—transitions. For young people who are enamored with routines and sameness, as are many individuals with autism spectrum disorder (ASD), the daily transitions of life can be overwhelming: The route taken to school. The route

[a] Neuropsychiatry Outpatient Program, Adult Developmental Neuropsychiatry Clinic, Adult Inpatient Intellectual Disability and Autism Unit, Sheppard Pratt Autism Registry, Ethics Committee, Sheppard Pratt Health System, 6501 North Charles Street, Baltimore, MD 21204, USA; [b] Adult Developmental Neuropsychiatry Clinic, Sheppard Pratt Health System, 6501 North Charles Street, Baltimore, MD 21204, USA; [c] Sheppard Pratt Health System, 6501 North Charles Street, Baltimore, MD 21204, USA
* Corresponding author.
E-mail address: rwisner-carlson@sheppardpratt.org

Child Adolesc Psychiatric Clin N Am 29 (2020) 345–358
https://doi.org/10.1016/j.chc.2019.12.002
1056-4993/20/© 2019 Elsevier Inc. All rights reserved.

taken home. The rituals that begin the day, continue the day, and end the day. A minor disruption in any of these can be a significant challenge to the person with ASD and their caretakers, potentially leading to upset, withdrawal, self-injurious behaviors, or aggression. The transition to adulthood for a person with ASD can be a period for growth or can completely derail their existence. Whether moving to supported day activities, employment, or higher education, young people with autism face significant and unique challenges. Because autism occurs at all levels of intelligence and functioning, the extent of these challenges will vary. The challenges and potential services to overcome them as revealed by the literature will be the focus of this and the following articles.

OUTCOMES AND THE EXTENT OF THE PROBLEM

Outcomes for individuals with ASD have improved since Kanner's 1943 landmark paper, "Autistic disturbances of affective contact,"[1] and continue to advance with more young adults with autism going to college and entering the workforce.[2] However, just as Kanner's patient Donald was underemployed, socially isolated, and continued to live with his parents in adulthood,[3] most young adults with ASD today face similar circumstances.[4] Overall, the literature for ASD in adulthood reflects poorer outcomes compared with neurotypical peers in terms of jobs, relationships, independent living, and mental health.[5]

Key findings of the *National Autism Indicators Report: Transition into Young Adulthood* in 2015 include the following:

- 58% of young adults with ASD worked for pay outside the home in the years after high school and tended to work part-time in low-wage jobs;
- 36% attended a 2-year or 4-year college or vocational education;
- Only 1 in 5 adults with ASD lived independently between high school and their early 20s;
- An estimated 1 in 4 young adults with autism were socially isolated, meaning "they never saw or talked with friends and were never invited to social activities within the past year"; and
- Approximately 26% of young adults on the autism spectrum received no services—services that could help them become employed, continue their education, or live more independently.[6]

For most young people, the transition to adulthood is both an exciting and stressful time. Classically, the task of this transition has been described by developmental psychologist Erik Erikson as mastering the challenge of intimacy versus isolation; this task coming after the adolescent task of identity versus role confusion.[7] More recently, Arnett and others have developed the concept of "emerging adulthood," a time of life from about 18 to 29 years of age in Western societies during which individuals are exploring various adult roles in work, relationships, and living situations. Emerging adulthood is a distinct new life stage created by the rise in the average age of marriage and parenthood since the middle of the twentieth century. Individuals in this stage are self-focused in exploring their identity and moving between adolescence and full adulthood, and are optimistic about the possibilities in their lives. There is considerable instability and change as these possibilities are explored. By the end of emerging adulthood, the individual accepts responsibility for one's self, makes decisions independently, and becomes financially independent, reaching full adulthood by the mid to late twenties.[8]

For their neurotypical peers traversing emerging adulthood, life is filled with possibilities, and this period is characterized by optimism: a period "when hope flourishes and people have an unparalleled opportunity to transform their lives."[8] Such optimism is less frequently present in young adults with ASD,[9] although this issue is complicated. Youth with ASD and their parents or caregivers experience fear and anxiety about transitioning to adulthood.[10] Caregiver burden is high during the transition to adolescence and adulthood, mainly because of unmet needs.[11] Parents of ASD individuals experience more distress after their child transitions out of high school.[12] A disparity in transition planning also may exist, with youth with ASD estimated to receive transition services half as often as youth with other special health care needs.[13] This disparity for transition planning is worse for ASD youth of racial/ethnic minorities or low-income families, and these individuals are yet more disconnected from educational, occupational, and social activities as they enter adulthood in comparison with their ASD peers without these added issues.[14] Individuals with ASD and their families are exposed to a "lifetime of difficult transitions." Owing to a lack of adequate resources in the adult transition period, ASD individuals and their families are concerned about being able to establish a meaningful adult life.[15]

Supporting these concerns, Quality of Life (QoL),[16–19] a concept that includes objective and subjective measures of health and functioning such as schooling, employment, and relationships, is much lower in individuals with ASD across the life span in comparison with their peers.[20] However, QoL and life satisfaction in ASD may be subjectively different from the perspective of the individual with autism. Egilson and colleagues[21] found that children with ASD report better QoL compared with the proxy reports of their parents. Cribb and colleagues[22] report a study of 26 young adults with ASD in emerging adulthood who describe feeling more in control of their lives as a result of the transition. These and other observations suggest that outcomes in the transition to adulthood for autistic individuals are complex and nuanced, and their life satisfaction may relate to outcomes and variables that are not fully appreciated by researchers.[23]

BURDENS AND BARRIERS TO TRANSITION

Individuals with ASD have a multitude of burdens causing difficulties in the transition to adulthood. Burdens range from those inherent in the condition, such as impaired social cognition and executive dysfunction, to identified cognitive issues/intellectual disability and comorbid medical and psychiatric diagnoses that occur at a higher rate for those with ASD.[24–27] Young adults with autism also face significant barriers to services at this time, such as a shortage of adult providers for psychiatric and medical issues and "a cliff of services" as they age out of childhood support.[28] To help manage this transition, psychiatrists and other health care providers must be aware of these issues and should aim to be helpful with community referrals.

A deficit in social communication and interaction is the hallmark of ASD.[29] Poor social skills affect one's ability to manage a life transition that requires meeting new people and developing relationships outside the family. Problems in social interactions may inhibit individuals in this population as they leave high school and move into other settings. There are new acquaintances such as classmates and employers to be met, new friends to be made, and likely less tolerance for what is perceived as social oddness and rude behavior. Remarks that may have been tolerated in the school classroom, where the autistic student's issues were well known and documented in an Individualized Education Plan, could lead to social ostracizing and work difficulties including loss of employment.[30] Underscoring this issue, a significant proportion of transition-age youth with ASD are socially isolated and become more so during the transition years.[31,32]

Executive function (EF) deficits also cause difficulties in the transition to adulthood. EF is an umbrella term referring to a set of abilities including forming goals, planning, carrying out goal-directed plans, mental flexibility, initiating action, and monitoring performance.[33,34] These cognitive processes are linked to frontal lobe activity and allow an individual to "filter...[information], engage in goal-directed behaviors, anticipate the consequences of one's actions and exhibit...mental flexibility."[35] EF is required for "appropriate, socially responsible, and effectively self-serving adult conduct."[36,p.666] Executive dysfunction is found in both neurologic (eg, traumatic brain injury, dementia, Korsakoff syndrome, progressive supranuclear palsy) and psychiatric (eg, attention deficit hyperactivity disorder, borderline personality disorder, substance abuse, schizophrenia) conditions,[35] including ASD.[37–41] EF impairments have been demonstrated in both children and adults with autism.[42–44]

In ASD, measures of EF earlier in life in a group of individuals with IQ higher than 70 predicted adaptive behaviors later in life.[45] This group included individuals as old as 23 years at follow-up. Childhood EF measures in a group of cognitively able children with ASD predicted adaptive behavior at 12-year follow-up.[46] In addition, EF explained adaptive behavior in a group of school-age youth with ASD and IQ lower than 75.[47] Impairment in EF has been linked to lower QoL in children with ASD.[48] It should be noted that adaptive function is lower than what would be expected for IQ in youth and adults with ASD as demonstrated with the Vineland II, a standard and widely used measure of adaptive function.[49] Adaptive functioning substantially lags behind IQ in young adulthood, and comorbid psychopathology significantly correlates with the size of IQ-adaptive functioning discrepancy.[50]

Deficits in EF are also thought to be involved in the deficits in social communication and interaction in individuals with ASD. EF deficits correlate with social functioning in elementary-school-aged children with ASD.[51] EF predicts the development of play skills for ASD preschoolers with verbal skills.[52] EF (initiation, working memory, planning, organization, and monitoring) effects social functioning in children and adolescents with ASD.[53] Theory of mind (ToM), the ability to attribute mental states to oneself and others, has also been connected with EF. Training EF in children with ASD improves performance on ToM tasks; however, training ToM does not improve performance on EF tasks.[54]

Thus, from the foregoing discussion, transition-age youth with ASD have weaknesses in social interactions, social cognition, and EF that will negatively affect their ability to enter the adult world. These young adults face difficulties managing their social life but also in planning, monitoring, and organizing the increasingly complex expectations and activities of their lives. At the same time, they are burdened with a greater likelihood of having medical and psychiatric conditions,[24–27] managing these conditions, and also transitioning to adult providers.[55–59]

THE ADULT WORLD

Key markers of the adult world include living independently from parents, financial independence, completing school, obtaining full-time employment, getting married, and becoming a parent.[60] Individuals with autism may need assistance navigating and achieving these milestones. This section discusses the challenges and related programs that may be available in the community.

Independent Living

Anderson and colleagues[61] analyzed data from the National Longitudinal Transition Study-2 (NLTS2). They found that young adults with ASD who are eligible for special education under the autism category are more likely to live with their parents or guardians and for longer periods of time after high school compared with individuals with other special education-defined disabilities (ie, mental retardation [intellectual disability], learning disabilities, emotional disturbances as per the Individuals with Disabilities Education Act). In addition, young adults with ASD are more likely to live in a supervised living arrangement and less likely to live independently in comparison with the other disability categories. This trend for low levels of independent living continues into adulthood for those with autism.[62] Various housing options outside the parental home may be available, from supported and supervised living situations, to group homes, to large residential programs, such as a residential farm. Funding may be an issue.[63]

Education

With improvements in ASD outcomes, more individuals with ASD are attending institutions of higher education. Autistic students preparing to start university express concerns about managing social, academic, and practical living domains, as well as the loss of home structure and the general transition to adulthood.[64] These concerns are validated by autistic individuals' reports of their college experiences. Overall, individuals with ASD report receiving academic support in college, although there is less attention to social and emotional domains.[65,66] Transitions are often unplanned, and disclosure of diagnosis uncommonly occurs after a significant problem.[66] Some students hesitate to use supporting services and disclose their disability, thus accessing less support and having a overall poorer university experience.[67] Autistic college students and their parents report the greatest struggles with social tasks and activities of daily living.[68] Poor emotional regulation also is regarded as an issue for support.[69]

The hesitancy to disclose the ASD diagnosis is understandable. In a study reported in 2011, typically developing college peers without a first-degree relative with an ASD diagnosis were significantly less open toward peers with ASD. It is hoped that, over the last decade, these views have evolved. A peer-mentoring program at a university in Australia improves ASD knowledge and is experienced as being overwhelmingly positive by the mentors.[70] University faculty feel insufficiently prepared to work with students with ASD, lack knowledge on accommodations, and are not proactive with providing accommodations in the classroom.[71]

Transition programs such as the Stepped Transition in Education Program for Students with ASD (STEPS)[72,73] and the Collaborative Model for Promoting Competence and Success (COMPASS)[74,75] have been developed to improve the transition from high school to college. Programs in college include those with a clinical focus, a social skills focus, and/or an academic focus, available at select colleges and universities.[76]

Employment

Adults with ASD have lower rates of employment and/or are underemployed, as documented in the National Autism Indicators Report. Competitive integrated employment success can be significantly improved with specific interventions including the transition to work internship program called Project SEARCH+ASD, supported employment, and other means. This aspect is reviewed in detail by Carol Schall and colleagues' article, "Competitive Integrated Employment for Youth and Adults with Autism: Findings from a Scoping Review," in this issue.

Driving

With ridesharing services such as Uber and Lyft and the promise of the future self-driving car, driving in American society may not remain the rite of passage from childhood into young adulthood it once was. However, transportation continues to be an important issue for individuals with ASD. When surveyed, young adults with ASD, in comparison with their typically developing peers, report less preference for driving, less confidence in their driving abilities, and more anxiety around driving.[77] Licensed adult drivers with ASD, completing the Driver Behavior Questionnaire, endorse lower ratings of their ability to drive and more traffic accidents and citations.[78]

Parents and caregivers of young adults with ASD indicate that learning to drive presents a substantial challenge. The complex demands of driving, including multi-tasking, are a particular problem.[79] In a study using the Driving Attitude Scale Parent-Report, parents of novice drivers with ASD report less positive and more negative attitudes of their ASD children compared with parents of neurotypical novice drivers. These attitudes could be improved by providing driver training in a low-threat virtual reality driving simulator.[80] Driving instructors in Belgium completing a driver instructor questionnaire advised an individual approach emphasizing structure, clarity, visual demonstration, practice, and repetition when teaching individuals with ASD to drive.[81]

Difficulties in driving have been measured in individuals with ASD. Research has suggested that adult men with ASD have more difficulty identifying social hazards compared with typically developing peers. Nonsocial hazard recognition was similar in the 2 groups.[82] However, more recent research has not fully supported this finding. Reaction times to social hazards for typically developing drivers were faster for social hazards than for nonsocial hazards. For ASD drivers, the reaction times were equal; this did not affect driving performance.[83] Assessment of driving simulator performance and EF in novice drivers with and without ASD showed poorer driving performance overall in the ASD group. Driving performance was worsened by a working memory task, more so for ASD compared with control drivers.[84]

As already indicated, surveyed driving instructors have recommended a more structured and individualized approach to driver training for individuals with ASD.[81] Other interventions include using a driving simulator to train the motor aspects of driving[85] and improving visual attention[86] in young ASD drivers, and the use of virtual reality driving paradigms for driver training.[87–90] Thus, learning to drive is exemplary of issues faced by individuals with ASD related to social cognition and EF deficits and the types of interventions that may help, including individualized support and technology.

Independent Life Skills

Independent life skills and adaptive behaviors, including activities of daily living such as hygiene and basic self-care as well as instrumental activities of daily living such as money management and driving, are vital for individuals with ASD during the transition to adulthood. Adaptive behaviors such as possessing functional communication, being able to take care of one's hygiene, and having meaningful relationships with others contribute to how well an individual is able to gain independence.[91] Studies have shown that low IQ and communication deficits lead to poorer outcomes in relation to independent life skills.[5] Likewise, individuals with high IQs may struggle with gaining independence if they possess deficits across adaptive behaviors.[91] Children with ASD show deficits across various daily living skills and, despite making some gains through adolescence, these skills tend to level out by young adulthood.[49,92]

Early intervention that focuses on enhancing cognitive and language skills as well as teaching daily life skills constitutes the first step in nurturing independence among individuals diagnosed with ASD.[49,92] Ongoing assessment of adaptive behaviors can help identify areas that are in need of improvement and help to identify goals that can be targeted across environments.[91,93] Speech and language pathologists can provide ongoing assessment of language ability and tailor a plan to help the individual to learn to communicate with others. Likewise, functional communication training could be implemented to effectively increase the individual's behavioral repertoire in verbalizing one's needs rather than engaging in inappropriate behaviors to realize that need.[94] Taking a more behavioral approach in training across verbal operants can also increase effective communication skills in individuals with ASD.[95] Further developing language in social settings can be facilitated via group social skills training[96] to help individuals interact with others. Finally, individuals must be able to generalize their communicative ability across environments and individuals, thus helping to facilitate independent living.

Likewise, daily life skills can be taught in person or through video instruction using modeling or via task analysis, a method of breaking down a task into simple steps.[97] For example, to learn how to brush one's teeth, a caregiver can identify all of the steps in performing such a task and assess how the individual with ASD completes each action associated with that task. Caregivers can then identify the deficits observed and focus training on those areas of weakness. Taken as a whole, individuals with ASD require additional support early on in learning how to perform daily life functions. Without these building blocks in place at an early age, an individual with ASD may find greater difficulty in gaining independent life skills as he or she transitions to adulthood.

Skill building must continue throughout early childhood and adolescence. Caregivers and teachers can continue building on previously mastered skills and create new objective goals to meet. Given that the learning of new skills tends to slow down significantly toward late adolescence, a focus on this time is necessary. Academic and career planning for individuals with ASD should begin early and before the individual has left secondary school.[93] Academic support should meet the needs of the individual and help in the continued development of adaptive skills necessary for independent living. Furthermore, including the individual in making future plans is important in fostering motivation to reach target goals.[93] Working toward developing independent life skills and obtaining individualized and increased support foster better academic[93] and career[98] performance which, in turn, helps reinforce and nurture independence.

Money Management

Being able to manage one's finances is essential to living an independent life. An individual must find a source of income, budget for necessary items and shelter, keep track of and balance finances, and have savings set aside for emergencies. Money management involves multiple components, and failure to do so effectively and efficiently can lead to dire consequences such as lack of shelter and reduced access to services and food. This can be a daunting task for anyone and can be especially difficult for individuals with ASD. The literature suggests that these individuals worry about their lack of being able to manage finances and see this as a barrier to becoming an independent adult.[99]

Individuals with ASD may require additional support with activities such as hygiene, communication, and other day-to-day tasks. Being able to manage one's finances is no exception, and should be assessed and taught throughout the life span. Prerequisites include being able to count money and determine whether one has enough to purchase an item or service. Training programs for individuals with ASD have been shown to effectively increase participants' ability to independently identify and count money and apply it to costing of an item in a contrived setting and later generalized out in the community.[100] Starting in adolescence, individuals with ASD must be taught more complicated financial management skills, including budgeting resources and accessing banking services. As these individuals emerge into adulthood, transition programs can be effective in identifying needs and providing additional support in helping them become more financially autonomous, which plays a larger role in being able to live independently as they grow older.[101]

SUMMARY

With nearly 1.7% of 8-year-old children in the United States now identified as having ASD by the Centers of Disease Control and Prevention, it is incumbent on all psychiatrists—child, adolescent, adult—to fully understand the special needs and services required by ASD youth and adults to succeed. The transition to adulthood for young people with autism is difficult because of the deficits in social cognition and EF that are inherent in the ASD diagnosis and serve as barriers to success during this critical phase of life. This difficulty is exacerbated by loss of services at a time when the complexity of expectations is increasing. Although more community-based services are available to help support individuals overcome these barriers, too many young people with autism are failing to achieve the milestones of adulthood, as evidenced by woefully unacceptable outcomes data. Social skills training, employment interventions, college transition programs, and driver training technologies are potential interventions to help those with ASD overcome the barriers. Over the last few decades, significant advances in early childhood interventions for ASD have led to more young adults with ASD in college and the workforce. Now these childhood interventions need to be followed by a range of best practices implemented for the transition to adulthood and beyond. Children with ASD grow up and this condition persists throughout the life span. These young people need to be connected to services that will allow them to thrive in adulthood. That is their hope and should be our goal as clinicians.

DISCLOSURE

The authors have nothing to disclose.

REFERENCES

1. Kanner L. Autistic disturbances of affective contact. Nervous child. Nerv Child 1943.
2. van Schalkwyk GI, Volkmar FR. Autism spectrum disorders: challenges and opportunities for transition to adulthood. Child Adolesc Psychiatr Clin N Am 2017. https://doi.org/10.1016/j.chc.2016.12.013.
3. Kanner L. Follow-up study of eleven autistic children originally reported in 1943. J Autism Child Schizophr 1995;1(2):119–45.
4. Newman L, Wagner M, Knokey AM, et al. The post-high school outcomes of young adults with disabilities up to 8 years after high school: a report from the National Longitudinal Transition Study-2 (NLTS2). NCSER 2011-3005, vol. 2. Washington, DC: National Center for Special Education Research; 2011. p. 218. Available at: https://ies.ed.gov/ncser/pubs/20113005/pdf/20113005.pdf.
5. Howlin P, Magiati I. Autism spectrum disorder: outcomes in adulthood. Curr Opin Psychiatry 2017;30(2):69–76.
6. Roux AM, Shattuck PT, Rava JE, et al. National autism indicators report: transition into young adulthood. Philadelphia (PA): AJ Drexel Autism Institute; 2015. Available at: https://iacc.hhs.gov/publications/general/2015/natl-autism-indicators-report-july-2015.pdf.
7. Erikson EH. Childhood and society. New York: WW Norton & Co; 1963.

8. Arnett JJ. Emerging adulthood: the winding road from the late teens through the twenties. New York: Oxford University Press; 2006. https://doi.org/10.1093/acprof:oso/9780195309379.001.0001.

9. Schmidt L, Kirchner J, Strunz S, et al. Psychosocial functioning and life satisfaction in adults with autism spectrum disorder without intellectual impairment. J Clin Psychol 2015;71(12):1259–68.

10. Cheak-Zamora NC, Teti M, First J. "Transitions are scary for our kids, and they're scary for us": family member and youth perspectives on the challenges of transitioning to adulthood with autism. J Appl Res Intellect Disabil 2015;28(6):548–60.

11. Cadman T, Eklund H, Howley D, et al. Caregiver burden as people with autism spectrum disorder and attention-deficit/hyperactivity disorder transition into adolescence and adulthood in the United Kingdom. J Am Acad Child Adolesc Psychiatry 2012;51(9):879–88.

12. McKenzie K, Ouellette-Kuntz H, Blinkhorn A, et al. Out of school and into distress: families of young adults with intellectual and developmental disabilities in transition. J Appl Res Intellect Disabil 2017;30(4):774–81.

13. Cheak-Zamora NC, Yang X, Farmer JE, et al. Disparities in transition planning for youth with autism spectrum disorder. Pediatrics 2013;131(3):447–54.

14. Eilenberg JS, Paff M, Harrison AJ, et al. Disparities based on race, ethnicity, and socioeconomic status over the transition to adulthood among adolescents and young adults on the autism spectrum: a systematic review. Curr Psychiatry Rep 2019;21(5). https://doi.org/10.1007/s11920-019-1016-1.

15. Milen MT, Nicholas DB. Examining transitions from youth to adult services for young persons with autism. Soc Work Health Care 2017;56(7):636–48.

16. Testa MA, Simonson DC. Assessment of quality-of-life outcomes. N Engl J Med 1996. https://doi.org/10.1056/NEJM199603283341306.

17. Jenkins C. Quality of life. Encylopaedia Britannica. 2019. Available at: https://www.britannica.com/topic/quality-of-life. Accessed August 25, 2019.

18. WHOQOL. Measuring quality of life. Available at: https://www.who.int/healthinfo/survey/whoqol-qualityoflife/en/. Accessed August 25, 2019.

19. The World Health Organization quality of life assessment (WHOQOL): position paper from the World Health Organization. Soc Sci Med 1995. https://doi.org/10.1016/0277-9536(95)00112-K.

20. Van Heijst BFC, Geurts HM. Quality of life in autism across the lifespan: a meta-analysis. Autism 2015;19(2):158–67.

21. Egilson ST, Ólafsdóttir LB, Leósdóttir T, et al. Quality of life of high-functioning children and youth with autism spectrum disorder and typically developing peers: self- and proxy-reports. Autism 2017;21(2):133–41.

22. Cribb S, Kenny L, Pellicano E. 'I definitely feel more in control of my life': the perspectives of young autistic people and their parents on emerging adulthood. Autism 2019. https://doi.org/10.1177/1362361319830029.

23. Henninger NA, Taylor JL. Outcomes in adults with autism spectrum disorders: a historical perspective. Autism 2013. https://doi.org/10.1177/1362361312441266.

24. Davignon MN, Qian Y, Massolo M, et al. Psychiatric and medical conditions in transition-aged individuals with ASD. Pediatrics 2018;141(April 2018):S335–45.

25. Lai M-C, Kassee C, Besney R, et al. Prevalence of co-occurring mental health diagnoses in the autism population: a systematic review and meta-analysis. Lancet Psychiatry 2019;6(10):819–29.

26. Mosner MG, Kinard JL, Shah JS, et al. Rates of co-occurring psychiatric disorders in autism spectrum disorder using the mini international neuropsychiatric interview. J Autism Dev Disord 2019;49(9):3819–32.

27. Rosen TE, Mazefsky CA, Vasa RA, et al. Co-occurring psychiatric conditions in autism spectrum disorder. Int Rev Psychiatry 2018;30(1):40–61.

28. Turcotte P, Mathew M, Shea LL, et al. Service needs across the lifespan for individuals with autism. J Autism Dev Disord 2016. https://doi.org/10.1007/s10803-016-2787-4.

29. American Psychiatric Association. Diagnostic and statistical manual of mental disorders. 5th edition. Arlington (VA): American Psychiatric Association; 2013.

30. Schall C, Wehman P, Carr S. Transition from high school to adulthood for adolescents and young adults with autism spectrum disorders. In: Volkmar FR, Reichow B, McPartland JC, editors. Adolescents and adults with autism spectrum disorders. New York: Springer; 2014. p. 41–60. https://doi.org/10.1007/978-1-4939-0506-5_3.

31. Liptak GS, Kennedy JA, Dosa NP. Social participation in a nationally representative sample of older youth and young adults with autism. J Dev Behav Pediatr 2011;32(4):277–83.

32. Orsmond GI, Shattuck PT, Cooper BP, et al. Social participation among young adults with an autism spectrum disorder. J Autism Dev Disord 2013. https://doi.org/10.1007/s10803-013-1833-8.

33. Jurado MB, Rosselli M. The elusive nature of executive functions: a review of our current understanding. Neuropsychol Rev 2007. https://doi.org/10.1007/s11065-007-9040-z.

34. Chan RCK, Shum D, Toulopoulou T, et al. Assessment of executive functions: review of instruments and identification of critical issues. Arch Clin Neuropsychol 2008;23(2):201–16.

35. Alfredo Ardela VWM. Executive dysfunction. Medlink neurology. 2018. Available at: https://www.medlink.com/article/executive_dysfunction. Accessed September 14, 2019.

36. Lezak MD, Howieson D, Bigler ED, et al. Neuropsychological assessment. 5th edition. New York: Oxford University Press; 2012. p. 2012.

37. Hughes C, Russell J, Robbins TW. Evidence for executive dysfunction in autism. Neuropsychologia 1994;32(4):477–92.

38. Robinson S, Goddard L, Dritschel B, et al. Executive functions in children with autism spectrum disorders. Brain Cogn 2009;71(3):362–8.

39. Hill EL. Executive dysfunction in autism. Trends Cogn Sci 2004;8(1):26–32.

40. Demetriou EA, Lampit A, Quintana DS, et al. Autism spectrum disorders: a meta-analysis of executive function. Mol Psychiatry 2018;23(5):1198–204.

41. McLean RL, Johnson Harrison A, Zimak E, et al. Executive function in probands with autism with average IQ and their unaffected first-degree relatives. J Am Acad Child Adolesc Psychiatry 2014;53(9):1001–9.

42. Bramham J, Ambery F, Young S, et al. Executive functioning differences between adults with attention deficit hyperactivity disorder and autistic spectrum disorder in initiation, planning and strategy formation. Autism 2009;13(3):245–64.

43. Davids RCD, Groen Y, Berg IJ, et al. Executive functions in older adults with autism spectrum disorder: objective performance and subjective complaints. J Autism Dev Disord 2016;46(9):2859–73.

44. Johnston K, Murray K, Spain D, et al. Executive function: cognition and behaviour in adults with Autism Spectrum Disorders (ASD). J Autism Dev Disord 2019; 2013. https://doi.org/10.1007/s10803-019-04133-7.

45. Pugliese CE, Anthony LG, Strang JF, et al. Longitudinal examination of adaptive behavior in autism spectrum disorders: influence of executive function. J Autism Dev Disord 2016;46(2):467–77.

46. Kenny L, Cribb SJ, Pellicano E. Childhood executive function predicts later autistic features and adaptive behavior in young autistic people: a 12-year prospective study. J Abnorm Child Psychol 2019;47(6):1089–99.

47. Bertollo JR, Yerys BE. More than IQ: executive function explains adaptive behavior above and beyond nonverbal IQ in youth with autism and lower IQ. Am J Intellect Dev Disabil 2019;124(3):191–205.

48. de Vries M, Geurts H. Influence of autism traits and executive functioning on quality of life in children with an autism spectrum disorder. J Autism Dev Disord 2015;45(9):2734–43.

49. Matthews NL, Malligo A, Smith CJ. Toward the identification of adaptive functioning intervention targets for intellectually-able, transition-aged youth with autism: an examination of caregiver responses on the Vineland-II. Autism Res 2017;10(12):2023–36.

50. Kraper CK, Kenworthy L, Popal H, et al. The gap between adaptive behavior and intelligence in autism persists into young adulthood and is linked to psychiatric co-morbidities. J Autism Dev Disord 2017;47(10):3007–17.

51. Freeman LMM, Locke J, Rotheram-Fuller E, et al. Brief report: examining executive and social functioning in elementary-aged children with autism. J Autism Dev Disord 2017. https://doi.org/10.1007/s10803-017-3079-3.

52. Faja S, Dawson G, Sullivan K, et al. Executive function predicts the development of play skills for verbal preschoolers with autism spectrum disorders. Autism Res 2016. https://doi.org/10.1002/aur.1608.

53. Leung RC, Vogan VM, Powell TL, et al. The role of executive functions in social impairment in Autism Spectrum Disorder. Child Neuropsychol 2016;22(3):336–44.

54. Geurts HM, de Vries M, van den Bergh SFWM. Executive functioning theory and autism. In: Goldstein S, Naglieri JA, editors. Handbook of executive functioning. New York: Springer New York; 2014. p. 121–41. https://doi.org/10.1007/978-1-4614-8106-5_8.

55. Hall T, Kriz D, Duvall S, et al. Healthcare transition challenges faced by young adults with autism spectrum disorder. Clin Pharmacol Ther 2015;98(6):573–5.

56. Kuhlthau KA, Delahaye J, Erickson-Warfield M, et al. Health care transition services for youth with Autism Spectrum Disorders: perspectives of caregivers. Pediatrics 2016;137(3):S158–66.

57. Cheak-Zamora NC, Teti M, Maurer-Batjer A, et al. Exploration and comparison of adolescents with autism spectrum disorder and their caregiver's perspectives on transitioning to adult health care and adulthood. J Pediatr Psychol 2017; 42(9):1028–39.

58. Cheak-Zamora NC, Farmer JE, Mayfield WA, et al. Health care transition services for youth with autism spectrum disorders. Rehabil Psychol 2014. https://doi.org/10.1037/a0036725.

59. Walsh C, Jones B, Schonwald A. Health care transition planning among adolescents with autism spectrum disorder. J Autism Dev Disord 2017;47(4):980–91.

60. Scales PC, Benson PL, Oesterle S, et al. The dimensions of successful young adult development: a conceptual and measurement framework. Appl Dev Sci 2016;20(3):150–74.

61. Anderson KA, Shattuck PT, Cooper BP, et al. Prevalence and correlates of post-secondary residential status among young adults with an autism spectrum disorder. Autism 2014. https://doi.org/10.1177/1362361313481860.

62. Farley M, Cottle KJ, Bilder D, et al. Mid-life social outcomes for a population-based sample of adults with ASD. Autism Res 2018;11(1):142–52.

63. Atsmon T, Yaakobi L, Lowinger S. Adults on the autism spectrum and their families: residential issues. In: Lowinger S, Pearlman-Avnion S, editors. Autism in adulthood. 2019. p. 155–81. https://doi.org/10.1007/978-3-030-28833-4_8.

64. Lambe S, Russell A, Butler C, et al. Autism and the transition to university from the student perspective. Autism 2019;23(6):1531–41.

65. Gelbar NW, Shefcyk A, Reichow B. A comprehensive survey of current and former college students with autism. Yale J Biol Med 2015;88:45–68.

66. Cai RY, Richdale AL. Educational experiences and needs of higher education students with autism spectrum disorder. J Autism Dev Disord 2016;46(1):31–41.

67. Anderson AH, Carter M, Stephenson J. Perspectives of university students with autism spectrum disorder. J Autism Dev Disord 2018;48(3):651–65.

68. Elias R, White SW. Autism goes to college: understanding the needs of a student population on the rise. J Autism Dev Disord 2018. https://doi.org/10.1007/s10803-017-3075-7.

69. White SW, Elias R, Salinas CE, et al. Students with autism spectrum disorder in college: results from a preliminary mixed methods needs analysis. Res Dev Disabil 2016. https://doi.org/10.1016/j.ridd.2016.05.010.

70. Hamilton J, Stevens G, Girdler S. Becoming a mentor: the impact of training and the experience of mentoring university students on the autism spectrum. PLoS One 2016;11(4):e0153204.

71. Zeedyk SM, Bolourian Y, Blacher J. University life with ASD: faculty knowledge and student needs. Autism 2019;23(3):726–36.

72. White SW, Elias R, Capriola-Hall NN, et al. Development of a college transition and support program for students with autism spectrum disorder. J Autism Dev Disord 2017;47(10). https://doi.org/10.1007/s10803-017-3236-8.

73. White SW, Smith IC, Miyazaki Y, et al. Improving transition to adulthood for students with autism: a randomized controlled trial of STEPS. J Clin Child Adolesc Psychol 2019. https://doi.org/10.1080/15374416.2019.1669157.

74. Ruble L, McGrew JH, Snell-Rood C, et al. Adapting COMPASS for youth with ASD to improve transition outcomes using implementation science. Sch Psychol Q 2018;34(2):187–200.

75. Ruble LA, McGrew JH, Toland M, et al. Randomized control trial of COMPASS for improving transition outcomes of students with autism spectrum disorder. J Autism Dev Disord 2018;48(10):3586–95.

76. Brown JT, Wolf LE, Kroesser S. Innovative programming to support college students with autism spectrum disorders. In: Volkmar FR, Reichow B, McPartland JC, editors. Adolescents and adults with autism spectrum disorders. New York: Springer; 2014. p. 121–30. https://doi.org/10.1007/978-1-4939-0506-5_7.

77. Chee DYT, Lee HCY, Falkmer M, et al. Viewpoints on driving of individuals with and without autism spectrum disorder. Dev Neurorehabil 2015;18(1):26–36.

78. Daly BP, Nicholls EG, Patrick KE, et al. Driving behaviors in adults with autism spectrum disorders. J Autism Dev Disord 2014;44(12):3119–28.

79. Cox NB, Reeve RE, Cox SM, et al. Brief report: driving and young adults with ASD: parents' experiences. J Autism Dev Disord 2012;42(10):2257–62.

80. Ross V, Cox DJ, Reeve R, et al. Measuring the attitudes of novice drivers with autism spectrum disorder as an indication of apprehensive driving: going beyond basic abilities. Autism 2018;22(1):62–9.

81. Ross V, Jongen EMM, Vanvuchelen M, et al. Exploring the driving behavior of youth with an autism spectrum disorder: a driver instructor questionnaire. 2015 Driving Assessment Conference. Snowbird, Salt Lake City, Utah, June 22-25, 2015; 98–104. doi:10.17077/drivingassessment.1557

82. Sheppard E, Ropar D, Underwood G, et al. Brief report: driving hazard perception in autism. J Autism Dev Disord 2010;40(4):504–8.

83. Bishop HJ, Biasini FJ, Stavrinos D. Social and non-social hazard response in drivers with autism spectrum disorder. J Autism Dev Disord 2017;47(4):905–17.

84. Cox SM, Cox DJ, Kofler MJ, et al. Driving simulator performance in novice drivers with autism spectrum disorder: the role of executive functions and basic motor skills. J Autism Dev Disord 2016;46(4):1379–91.

85. Brooks J, Kellett J, Seeanner J, et al. Training the motor aspects of pre-driving skills of young adults with and without autism spectrum disorder. J Autism Dev Disord 2016;46(7):2408–26.

86. Wade J, Weitlauf A, Broderick N, et al. A pilot study assessing performance and visual attention of teenagers with ASD in a novel adaptive driving simulator. J Autism Dev Disord 2017;47(11):3405–17.

87. Wade J, Zhang L, Bian D, et al. A gaze-contingent adaptive virtual reality driving environment for intervention in individuals with autism spectrum disorders. ACM Trans Interact Intell Syst 2016;6(1). https://doi.org/10.1145/2892636.

88. Bian D, Wade J, Swanson A, et al. Physiology-based affect recognition during driving in virtual environment for autism intervention.. In: Placido da Silva H, Chauvet P, Holzinger A, et al, editors. PhyCS 2015: proceedings of the 2nd international conference on physiological computing systems. Portugal: SCITEPRESS; 2015. p. 137–45. https://doi.org/10.5220/0005331301370145.

89. Bian D, Wade J, Warren Z, et al. Online engagement detection and task adaptation in a virtual reality based driving simulator for autism intervention. In: Antona N, Stephanidis C, editors. UAHCI 2016: Universal access in human-computer interaction. Users and context diversity. Cham (Switzerland): Springer; 2016. p. 538–47.

90. Zhang L, Wade J, Bian D, et al. Multimodal fusion for cognitive load measurement in an adaptive virtual reality driving task for autism intervention. In: Antona N, Stephanidis C, editors. UAHCI 2015: Universal access in human-computer interaction. Access to learning, health and well-being. Cham (Switzerland): Springer; 2015. p. 709–20. https://doi.org/10.1007/978-3-319-20684-4_68.

91. Wise EA, Smith MD, Rabins PV. Correlates of daily functioning in older adults with autism spectrum disorder. Aging Ment Health 2019;1–9. https://doi.org/10.1080/13607863.2019.1647138.

92. Bal VH, Kim SH, Cheong D, et al. Daily living skills in individuals with autism spectrum disorder from 2 to 21 years of age. Autism 2015. https://doi.org/10.1177/1362361315575840.

93. Carter EW, Harvey MN, Taylor JL, et al. Connecting youth and young adults with autism spectrum disorders to community life. Psychol Sch 2013. https://doi.org/10.1002/pits.21716.

94. Mancil GR. Functional communication training: a review of the literature related to children with autism. Educ Train Dev Disabil 2006;41(3):213–24.

95. Sundberg ML, Michael J. The benefits of Skinner's analysis of verbal behavior for children with autism. Behav Modif 2001. https://doi.org/10.1177/0145445501255003.

96. Deckers A, Muris P, Roelofs J, et al. A group-administered social skills training for 8- to 12- year-old, high-functioning children with autism spectrum disorders: an evaluation of its effectiveness in a naturalistic outpatient treatment setting. J Autism Dev Disord 2016. https://doi.org/10.1007/s10803-016-2887-1.

97. Ayres KM, Maguire A, McClimon D. Acquisition and generalization of chained tasks taught with computer based video instruction to children with autism. Educ Train Dev Disabil 2009;44(4):493–508.

98. Hendricks D. Employment and adults with autism spectrum disorders: challenges and strategies for success. J Vocat Rehabil 2010. https://doi.org/10.3233/JVR-2010-0502.

99. Cheak-Zamora NC, Teti M, Peters C, et al. Financial capabilities among youth with autism spectrum disorder. J Child Fam Stud 2017;26(5):1310–7.

100. Cihak DF, Grim J. Teaching students with autism spectrum disorder and moderate intellectual disabilities to use counting-on strategies to enhance independent purchasing skills. Res Autism Spectr Disord 2008. https://doi.org/10.1016/j.rasd.2008.02.006.

101. Ross J, Marcell J, Williams P, et al. Postsecondary education employment and independent living outcomes of persons with autism and intellectual disability. J Postsecond Educ Disabil 2013;26(4):337–51.

Social Skills Training in Autism Spectrum Disorder Across the Lifespan

Christine T. Moody, MA*, Elizabeth A. Laugeson, PsyD[1]

KEYWORDS

- Autism spectrum disorder • Social skills • Social skills training • Lifespan
- Intervention

KEY POINTS

- Findings from the current literature review indicate that social skills training programs for individuals with autism spectrum disorder are effective in improving social competence, although effects are frequently not robust across all outcomes measured.
- When aggregating across the social skills training programs with the strongest evidence, common elements can be identified in both the treatment delivery method and the social skills content targeted.
- However, social skills training programs continue to remain limited in their generalizability and scope. Existing research has primarily tested programs designed for school-aged children with autism spectrum disorder, who have average or above average intellectual functioning.

The construct of social skills is both multidimensional and related to many other important constructs of interest, including cognition, language, and mental health. Despite this complexity, consensus in both colloquial and scholarly definitions of social skills involves common threads. Specifically, various definitions agree that social skills are socially acceptable, learned behaviors that enable individuals to function competently in various social tasks.[1] These specific behaviors, or skills, increase the likelihood of others receiving an individual positively and can be culturally bound.[2,3]

Using this definition, it is clear that social skills permeate successful adaptation in the development of positive personal relationships with family, friends, peers, and romantic partners.[4,5] However, social skills are also more broadly relevant to educational, professional, and daily living contexts whereby such skills are essential to effectively navigate complex interactions and group dynamics (eg, negotiating salaries, collaborating on school projects, living with roommates). Accordingly, teachers rate social skills as essential to children's success in the classroom,[6] and economists

University of California, Los Angeles, Los Angeles, CA, USA
[1] Present address: 300 Medical Plaza, Suite 1271, Los Angeles, CA 90095.
* Corresponding author. 1285 Franz Hall, Box 951563, Los Angeles, CA 90095.
E-mail address: christinemoody@ucla.edu

Child Adolesc Psychiatric Clin N Am 29 (2020) 359–371
https://doi.org/10.1016/j.chc.2019.11.001
1056-4993/20/© 2019 Elsevier Inc. All rights reserved.
childpsych.theclinics.com

document the value of social skills in predicting both employment and wages in young adulthood.[7]

Following from this, social skills consistently predict multiple important outcomes in the general population, including quality of life, self-esteem, and overall happiness. Research has further identified that the relationship between social skills and these outcomes is mediated by positive personal relationships.[8,9] Reciprocal friendships represent one such form of a positive personal relationship and provide protective effects against internalizing symptoms and maladjustment.[10,11] For youth, in particular, having even just one close friend can buffer against the negative sequelae of internalizing disorders[12,13] and peer victimization.[14]

SOCIAL SKILLS DEFICITS IN AUTISM SPECTRUM DISORDER

Despite their importance, there is significant individual variability in the mastery of social skills in children and adults. Autism spectrum disorder (ASD) is diagnostically characterized by deficits in social communication.[15] Social skill deficits in ASD are apparent in early childhood. Children with ASD show impairments in early communication, social attention, and pretend play skills.[16,17] Following this impaired social learning in early childhood, differences in the maturation of social behavior continue through developmental cascades.[18] Although the social communication deficits present in ASD are wide ranging and individuals vary broadly in their clinical presentation, pragmatic language deficits are considered to be universally present.[19] Pragmatic language, or the social use of language, encompasses skills, such as topic initiation and maintenance, turn-taking in conversation, providing the appropriate level of information, understanding nonliteral language, and appropriate modulation of communication based on context.[20]

Similar to the general population, research evidence suggests that these social skill deficits significantly interfere with the adjustment of individuals with ASD. Children with ASD, regardless of cognitive ability, are reported to have fewer friends and are less actively engaged in their social settings.[21,22] In adolescents and adults with ASD, greater social skills impairments predicted lower rates of social participation, with more than half of young adults with ASD reporting no close friendships.[23–25] Romantic relationships are impacted as well, with adults with ASD demonstrating inferior social knowledge and skills related to sexuality, privacy, and courting as compared with typically developing young adults.[26] Outside of relational outcomes, social skill deficits have been associated with poor academic performance[27] and poor employment outcomes in individuals with ASD.[28,29] Furthermore, these difficulties in navigating the social world have also been found to correspond to increased mental health problems in individuals with ASD.[30,31]

SOCIAL SKILLS TRAINING

Clearly, targeting social skills deficits in individuals with ASD is a critical path through which to improve outcomes in this population. Although typically developing individuals may intuitively learn social norms and skills, the impaired social learning common in ASD likely interferes with this normative process. Social skills training programs seek to remedy this gap by providing specific guidance into and knowledge of the social world. Although social skills training is a common intervention for children with ASD, there has been a historical lack of research evidence on its efficacy. In published articles searched through 2011, a high-quality review identified only 5 randomized controlled trials (RCTs) that tested social skills training groups in ASD populations, across all ages.[32] Those 5 studies provided preliminary support that social skills training groups can reduce loneliness and produce positive impacts on social competence and social functioning.

That being said, increasing scientific attention in the last decade has bolstered the evidence base of social skills training approaches. A more recent review and metaanalysis yielded 19 RCTs.[33] Synthesis analyses suggested an overall medium effect size of social skills training on social competence, with significant effects present in parent-report, self-report, observer-report, and task-based measures. However, positive effects of social skills training were not observed when using teacher-report as an outcome, and the effects in self-report appeared to be driven largely by changes in social skill knowledge, rather than changes in social behavior.[33] These results suggest that although the current state of the evidence supports the effectiveness of social skills training for mitigating the social deficits present in ASD, individuals with ASD may also need additional supports in enacting and generalizing social knowledge across environments. It is also possible that changes in social knowledge immediately following social skills training interventions generate downstream effects in social behavior, because skills are used and subsequently socially reinforced over time and across contexts. In support of the latter explanation, 2 studies do suggest that gains maintain, and for some outcomes improve further, over follow-up periods.[34,35]

Another metaanalysis examining only group social skills interventions for higher functioning individuals with ASD that used standardized measures of either autism-related social deficits (Social Responsiveness Scale; SRS-2)[36] or overall social skills (Social Skills Rating System; SSRS)[37] identified 8 RCTs.[38] Group social skills training interventions reliably produced changes in SRS total score, SRS subscale scores, and SSRS social skills subscale, with moderate to large effect sizes.[38] Moderator analyses suggested that social skills groups that included a concurrent parent group resulted in larger improvements on the SRS. Furthermore, more intense interventions in terms of time and dosage produced greater gains.

Ultimately, social skills training has been classified as an evidence-based practice for individuals with ASD.[39] However, the state of the evidence and the nature of the interventions vary across developmental stages. For example, for children in preschool and elementary school, play is the primary social context, and thus, play-based social skills are frequent targets of social skills training programs at this age. In contrast, at later developmental stages, conversations become the primary social context. Furthermore, most research studies examining social skills training have focused on elementary school-aged children with ASD, creating less thorough and rigorous evidence for social skills training for other age groups. The following sections seek to review the research evidence for social skills training across 4 developmental stages: early childhood, elementary school, adolescence, and adulthood. For conciseness, the review primarily focuses on RCTs, which are considered the gold standard for assessing treatment outcome.

REVIEW OF RESEARCH EVIDENCE
Early Childhood (0–6 years)

Although autism symptoms and associated social deficits can be detected as early as 12 months of age, few social skills training programs for very young children with ASD have been systematically tested. A review of social skills interventions for this age range found that most eligible studies (31 of 35) were single-subject designs.[40] Definably, social skills training in this age range is also less clear than at later developmental stages. Specifically, interventions at this age may aim to produce gains in a child's receptive and expressive language, a domain that is intertwined but distinct from social skills. Furthermore, some treatment approaches emphasize prelinguistic social skills, such as joint attention, and naturalistic play interactions in order to promote normalized social attention and engagement as a way to alter the social trajectories of young children with ASD.[41] In contrast, traditional social skills training interventions represent an alternative path to learning social skills through direct teaching of social behavior and explicit rehearsal. As such, although these naturalistic developmental behavioral interventions may be effective for enhancing certain social skills in preschoolers with ASD,[41] they fall out of the scope of this review on social skills training.

In general, preliminary evidence suggests that social skills training groups can be effective in early childhood development. In 1 study of 4 to 6 year olds with ASD, a social skills group used video modeling of typical peers enacting specific skills paired with play activities to practice and reinforce modeled skills.[42] A variety of play-related skills (eg, imitation, turn taking, seeking play partners) and social engagement skills (eg, eye contact, social smile) were taught. This intervention group was compared with an active control group of children with ASD who participated in free play with minimal socialization guidance. Relative to this free play group, children in the direct teaching group showed significant increases in social initiation, responding, and interacting behaviors with peers.[42] In another RCT, a social skills training group called Peer Networks intervention for 5 to 6 year olds with ASD was implemented in the school setting.[43] This treatment targeted requesting and sharing play objects, commenting on one's own play, commenting on others' play, good manners (eg, saying please, thank you), and common play rules. Skills were first taught through didactic instruction, followed by multiple role-play practices with feedback and a generalization play activity with peers. As compared with a treatment as usual group, children in Peer Networks showed more initiation with peers during generalization probes and greater social communication growth as reported by teachers, but no differences in social responses or total communication with peers.[43] In addition, Treatment and Education of Autistic and Communication related handicapped Children (TEACCH), which is an evidence-based program for individuals with ASD across the spectrum, tested a social skills training group for 5 to 6 year olds with ASD and average intellectual functioning. This program showed improved child social-emotional functioning and reduced parenting stress against a waitlist control group[44]; however, like many social skills treatment studies, this study was limited by its small sample size (n = 11).

Elementary School (7–12 years)

School-aged children have historically been the target population for social skills training programs. As such, there are numerous RCTs in this developmental stage, not all of which can be reviewed in depth in this article. Instead, the current review draws information from the most recent evidence syntheses. In the most recent comprehensive metaanalyses,[33,38] more than half of the included RCTs were tested in school-aged children with ASD. Both metaanalyses suggest that social skills training in this age range produces significant positive results in terms of social outcomes. All studies for school-aged children with ASD included in these metaanalyses used a small group format, although there was variability in the frequency and intensity of sessions. Several programs used a traditional 60- to 90-minute weekly session format,[45–48] whereas others implemented high-intensity programs using a summer camp format.[49–51] Despite these differences, the programs generally incorporated similar content, including emotion and facial expression recognition, body boundaries, responding to teasing, nonliteral language, perspective taking, and basic conversation skills (eg, listening, taking turns). Less common but still present were skills related to play and playdates, such as entering a group game, suggesting a change in play activity, and ways to maximize playdate success.[46] Concurrent parent training components were also frequently included for social skills training programs targeting school-aged children.

Adolescence (12–17 years)

Among the adolescent population, one of the most extensively tested social skills training programs for youth with ASD is the Program for the Education and Enrichment of Relational Skills (PEERS).[52] This program is characterized by 2 concurrent groups: a group for adolescents, in which the concrete rules of social skills are taught and practiced, and a parent group, in which parents are taught how to socially coach their adolescents in using the skills. Content includes conversational skills, appropriate use of humor, electronic communication, responding to bullying, good sportsmanship, and handling disagreements. In separate RCTs conducted by the treatment developers, PEERS for Adolescents produced social skills gains across a variety of measures, including standardized questionnaire assessment of overall social skills on SRSS, overall ASD symptoms related to social responsiveness on SRS, social knowledge, and number of hosted get-togethers with peers.[53,54] Furthermore, PEERS for Adolescents has been successfully adapted and replicated in multiple countries outside of North America, including South Korea,[55] Hong Kong,[56] and Israel.[57] Outside of social skill gains, multiple independent studies have found complementary benefits of the program to adolescents' mental health symptoms[58,59] and family stress.[60] Investigations into moderators of PEERS treatment outcome have suggested that the program is equally effective for male and female adolescents, as well as across early, middle, and late adolescence.[61,62]

Another social skills training program known as Multimodal Anxiety and Social Skills Intervention (MASSI) also found positive treatment results for adolescents with ASD as compared with waitlist controls in an RCT.[63] With its dual targets of anxiety and social deficits, MASSI combines multiple modalities, including individual therapy, a skills group, parent psychoeducation, and feedback from typically developing peers. Modules in individual therapy and in the skills group covered social skills content, including conversation skills, peer entry, and handling rejection, while weekly homework assignments were given to assist in mastery and generalization. Relative to the waitlist controls, social deficits as a function of autism symptoms decreased on the SRS in the active treatment group; however, anxiety symptoms did not differ between the treatment and control groups.

Although treatment outcomes appear encouraging for higher functioning adolescents with ASD, both PEERS and MASSI listed intellectual disability (ID) as an exclusionary criterion in their RCTs. Generally, very few social skills training programs are designed for the needs of individuals with ASD and comorbid ID. A review of literature in this area identified only 17 studies that targeted social behavior in primarily adolescents with ASD and ID; however, most were single-case research designs, frequently with idiosyncratic behavioral outcomes, thus, limiting conclusions about the efficacy of social skills training methods in this population.[64] Among adolescents with ASD and comorbid ID, behavioral teaching methods appeared to be the most effective in producing behavioral change in social behaviors.[64] More recently, video modeling has also been successfully applied and replicated as a method to teach specific social skills to adolescents with ASD and ID.[65,66]

Adulthood (18 years and Older)

Despite significant contextual changes in adulthood that might indicate a need for social skills training, particularly in relation to romantic relationships, workplace interactions, and independent living, few social skills programs exist for adults with ASD. With the strongest evidence, 3 RCTs of the PEERS for Young Adults program[67] have been conducted for young adults (18–24 years old) with ASD and without comorbid ID.[34,68,69] Structurally similar to the PEERS for Adolescents program, this program teaches skills through didactic instruction and uses a concurrent group of social coaches (eg, parents, life coaches, peer mentors) to provide support and performance feedback in naturalistic social settings. The content of the young adult program is similar to that of adolescents, with the significant addition of 4 sessions on dating skills. Findings from these RCTs support that, as compared with waitlist control groups, the PEERS for Young Adults program produces improvements in overall social skills and social responsiveness on standardized measures as well as increases in social skills knowledge, empathy, and social engagement.

Two other group designs tested interventions focused on vocational social skills. The Acquiring Career, Coping, Executive function, and Social Skills (ACCESS) program taught coping techniques, workplace social dynamics, building social support networks outside of the family, and self-determination skills, such as self-advocacy.[70] As compared with a waitlist control group, the young adults with ASD who received ACCESS showed significant gains in global adaptive functioning, although direct changes in social functioning were less pronounced.[70] In another study, a curriculum specific to social skills relevant to job interviewing demonstrated specific improvements on individuals' mock job interview performance, but participants did not show improvements on other standardized outcomes.[71] Both of these intervention protocols included direct teaching, role plays, and practicing of skills. ACCESS additionally incorporated weekly homework assignments and a concurrent social coach group for parents and other caregivers.

Recently, researchers have also begun to examine virtual reality platforms as a way to provide social skills training to higher-functioning adults with ASD. In 1 such study, a virtual reality platform was used specifically to target social skills needed during job interviews, such as sharing things in a positive way, conveying oneself professionally, negotiation, and building rapport with the interviewer.[72] The 10-hour virtual reality job interview training program offered specific guidance on the relevant social skills, in vivo coaching feedback through the platform, and multiple opportunities to rehearse interview skills. Young adults with ASD in the virtual reality job interview training program showed greater improvements in their live role-playing performance of an interview than young adults in the treatment as usual group.[72] Six months later, the group that received the virtual reality interview training was also significantly more likely to be competitively employed.[73]

SUMMARY

Social skills training programs are available for those with ASD from early childhood to young adulthood, with supporting evidence from multiple RCTs. Metaanalyses and systematic reviews continually support social skills training as efficacious in ameliorating social skills deficits in ASD.[32,33,38] Despite this, the density and quality of the evidence within the highlighted developmental groups vary. Overall, most of the research included in the current review was published within the last decade, signifying a significant increase in the evidence for social skills training programs for use with individuals with ASD.

Importantly, commonalities can be drawn from the current evidence base as to what works to produce meaningful change in the social outcomes of individuals with ASD. **Figs. 1** and **2** detail the emergent themes of effective intervention elements and

Program Structure	**In-Session Elements**	**Generalization Supports**
• Small group modality • Multiple staff • Routine session format • Concurrent parent training or peer involvement	• Didactic instruction of concrete skills • Modeling of skills • Skills practice with in vivo coaching feedback • Positive reinforcement (eg, praise, rewards)	• Homework assignments to practice skills in naturalistic settings • Parent or peer coaching outside of sessions to enhance generalization

Fig. 1. Common programmatic elements in evidence-based social skills training interventions for ASD.

content, respectively, in social skills training for ASD populations. Importantly, these figures are not representative of every *possible* effective intervention technique or helpful content area, but instead, document the methods and content that have generally been used in programs that produce clinically significant social gains. Many of the extracted commonalities are similar to previous summaries of components in evidence-based social skills training,[74,75] providing additional support for their validity. However, because the field is continuing to expand rapidly, updated reviews and syntheses will be needed in the coming years.

The common treatment elements used within evidence-based social skills training interventions generally draw from cognitive behavioral therapy (CBT) principles.[76] For example, psychoeducation, role-playing demonstrations, behavioral rehearsal, and

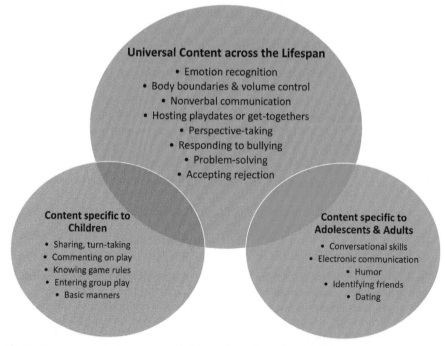

Fig. 2. Common content areas provided in evidence-based social skills training interventions for ASD.

homework assignments are common in CBT approaches. Many elements are also aligned with applied behavioral analysis (ABA), a core component of early intervention services for children with ASD.[77] In vivo coaching and performance feedback, positive reinforcement, and opportunities for generalization are all consistent with ABA.

FUTURE DIRECTIONS

Although the current literature provides evidence for the effectiveness of social skills training in individuals with ASD, more research is needed to confidently determine the efficacy, generalizability, and maintenance of treatment response to these approaches. In particular, future research would benefit from increased methodological rigor, through the following:

- Recruitment of larger sample sizes
- Utilization of active treatment controls
- Blind standardized assessment of outcome (eg, reduced reliance on parent- and self-report)
- Implementation of follow-up assessments to assess maintenance over time

All of these avenues of study are essential; however, the utilization of active treatment controls might be particularly pertinent. As most of the RCTs included in this review used a waitlist control group, it is possible that other mechanisms are accounting for treatment gains, such as group member interactions or therapeutic alliance. Ashman and colleagues[78] recently tested a didactic social skills training protocol against an active control group that facilitated positive social interactions among young adult participants through guided activities (eg, playing charades, discussing emotions in music). Both groups showed improvements over time, with no significant differences between them.[78] Similarly, a support group focused on social skills topics, which allowed groups of young adults with ASD to share their experiences and discuss solutions with little guidance, also resulted in increased empathy and fewer internalizing symptoms.[79] These findings lend some credence to the possibility that some of the positive effects observed in social skills training programs are due to nonspecific treatment factors.

In addition, studies in this field have neglected large swaths of individuals on the autism spectrum. As such, the research evidence is currently limited in its generalizability. In particular, there are gaps in the development and testing of social skills intervention for the following:

- Very young children (ie, 2–5 years old) with ASD
- Adults with ASD, especially middle-aged (ie, 35–55 years old) and older adults (ie, 55+ years old)
- Individuals with ASD struggling within specific social landscapes of adulthood (eg, vocational skills, romantic relationships, living outside of the home)
- Individuals with ASD and comorbid ID, across the lifespan
- Culturally and ethnically diverse individuals with ASD

Although some of these gaps have isolated exemplars of research teams investing implementation of social skills training in these groups, the scale of the need for services in these populations vastly outweighs the current evidence-based offerings.

Beyond increasing confidence in the current approaches, investigations into the moderators and mechanisms of treatment effects would be clinically useful. Furthermore, dismantling studies could elucidate the most essential pieces of the interventions, while augmentations to current evidence-based treatments could be tested as potential ways to strengthen gains. For example, extended length of programs with additional opportunities for skills practice could be tested against currently established treatments to determine if changes in dose result in greater gains. Ways to maximize cost-effectiveness and service reach while maintaining treatment efficacy could be explored as well, through group telehealth approaches or varying the size of the groups (eg, comparing a 6-person group to a 12-person group). In conclusion, although the evidence base for social skills training in ASD across the lifespan has grown significantly in the past decade, there is much yet to be developed and tested in order to improve the lives and enhance the social world of those with ASD.

DISCLOSURE

Dr. E.A. Laugeson receives royalties for book sales of PEERS manuals through Routledge; these manuals are referenced in the current article.

REFERENCES

1. Little SG, Swangler J, Akin-Little A. Defining social skills. In: Matson J, editor. Handbook of social behavior and skills in children. Cham (Switzerland): Springer International Publishing; 2017. p. 9–17.
2. Gresham FM, Elliott SN. Assessment and classification of children's social skills: a review of methods and issues. Sch Psychol Rev 1984;13(3):292–301.
3. Ladd GW. Children's peer relations and social competence: a century of progress. New Haven (CT): Yale University Press; 2005.
4. Crawford AM, Manassis K. Anxiety, social skills, friendship quality, and peer victimization: an integrated model. J Anxiety Disord 2011;25(7):924–31.
5. Engels RC, Finkenauer C, Meeus W, et al. Parental attachment and adolescents' emotional adjustment: the associations with social skills and relational competence. J Couns Psychol 2001;48(4):428–39.
6. Lane KL, Givner CC, Pierson MR. Teacher expectations of student behavior: social skills necessary for success in elementary school classrooms. J Spec Educ 2004;38(2):104–10.
7. Deming DJ. The growing importance of social skills in the labor market. Q J Econ 2017;132(4):1593–640.
8. Segrin C, Taylor M. Positive interpersonal relationships mediate the association between social skills and psychological well-being. Pers Individ Dif 2007;43(4):637–46.
9. Demir M, Jaafar J, Bilyk N, et al. Social skills, friendship and happiness: a cross-cultural investigation. J Soc Psychol 2012;152(3):379–85.
10. Bagwell CL, Kochel KP, Schmidt ME. Friendship and happiness in adolescence. In: Demir M, editor. Friendship and happiness. Dordrecht (the Netherlands): Springer; 2015. p. 99–116.
11. Waldrip AM, Malcolm KT, Jensen-Campbell LA. With a little help from your friends: the importance of high-quality friendships on early adolescent adjustment. Soc Dev 2008;17(4):832–52.
12. Erath SA, Flanagan KS, Bierman KL, et al. Friendships moderate psychosocial maladjustment in socially anxious early adolescents. J Appl Dev Psychol 2010; 31(1):15–26.
13. Kochel KP, Bagwell CL, Ladd GW, et al. Do positive peer relations mitigate transactions between depressive symptoms and peer victimization in adolescence? J Appl Dev Psychol 2017;51:44–54.

14. Rubin KH, Coplan R, Chen X, et al. Peer relationships in childhood. In: Lamb M, Bornstein M, editors. Social and personality development. New York: Psychology Press; 2013. p. 317–68.

15. American Psychiatric Association. Diagnostic and statistical manual of mental disorders. 5th Edition. Arlington (VA): American Psychiatric Association; 2013.

16. Ozonoff S, Iosif AM, Baguio F, et al. A prospective study of the emergence of early behavioral signs of autism. J Am Acad Child Adolesc Psychiatry 2010; 49(3):256–66.

17. Barbaro J, Dissanayake C. Autism spectrum disorders in infancy and toddlerhood: a review of the evidence on early signs, early identification tools, and early diagnosis. J Dev Behav Pediatr 2009;30(5):447–59.

18. Chevallier C, Kohls G, Troiani V, et al. The social motivation theory of autism. Trends Cogn Sci 2012;16(4):231–9.

19. Tager-Flusberg H, Paul R, Lord C. Language and communication in autism. In: Volkmar F, Paul R, Klin A, et al, editors. Handbook of autism and pervasive developmental disorders: diagnosis, development, neurobiology, and behavior. Hoboken (NJ): John Wiley & Sons, Inc; 2005. p. 335–64.

20. Volden J, Phillips L. Measuring pragmatic language in speakers with autism spectrum disorders: comparing the children's communication checklist—2 and the test of pragmatic language. Am J Speech Lang Pathol 2010;19(3):204–12.

21. Taheri A, Perry A, Minnes P. Examining the social participation of children and adolescents with intellectual disabilities and autism spectrum disorder in relation to peers. J Intellect Disabil Res 2016;60(5):435–43.

22. Kasari C, Locke J, Gulsrud A, et al. Social networks and friendships at school: comparing children with and without ASD. J Autism Dev Disord 2011;41(5): 533–44.

23. Orsmond GI, Krauss MW, Seltzer MM. Peer relationships and social and recreational activities among adolescents and adults with autism. J Autism Dev Disord 2004;34(3):245–56.

24. Eaves LC, Ho HH. Young adult outcome of autism spectrum disorders. J Autism Dev Disord 2008;38(4):739–47.

25. Howlin P, Goode S, Hutton J, et al. Adult outcome for children with autism. J Child Psychol Psychiatry 2004;45(2):212–29.

26. Stokes MA, Kaur A. High-functioning autism and sexuality: a parental perspective. Autism 2005;9(3):266–89.

27. Hsiao MN, Tseng WL, Huang HY, et al. Effects of autistic traits on social and school adjustment in children and adolescents: the moderating roles of age and gender. Res Dev Disabil 2013;34(1):254–65.

28. Chen JL, Leader G, Sung C, et al. Trends in employment for individuals with autism spectrum disorder: a review of the research literature. Rev J Autism Dev Disord 2015;2(2):115–27.

29. Chiang HM, Cheung YK, Li H, et al. Factors associated with participation in employment for high school leavers with autism. J Autism Dev Disord 2013; 43(8):1832–42.

30. Mayes SD, Calhoun SL, Murray MJ, et al. Variables associated with anxiety and depression in children with autism. J Dev Phys Disabil 2011;23(4):325–37.

31. Ratcliffe B, Wong M, Dossetor D, et al. The association between social skills and mental health in school-aged children with autism spectrum disorder, with and without intellectual disability. J Autism Dev Disord 2015;45(8):2487–96.

32. Reichow B, Steiner AM, Volkmar F. Cochrane review: social skills groups for people aged 6 to 21 with autism spectrum disorders (ASD). Evid Based Child Health 2013;8(2):266–315.

33. Gates JA, Kang E, Lerner MD. Efficacy of group social skills interventions for youth with autism spectrum disorder: a systematic review and meta-analysis. Clin Psychol Rev 2017;52:164–81.

34. Laugeson EA, Gantman A, Kapp SK, et al. A randomized controlled trial to improve social skills in young adults with autism spectrum disorder: the UCLA PEERS® program. J Autism Dev Disord 2015;45(12):3978–89.

35. Mandelberg J, Laugeson EA, Cunningham TD, et al. Long-term treatment outcomes for parent-assisted social skills training for adolescents with autism spectrum disorders: the UCLA PEERS program. J Ment Health Res Intellect Disabil 2014;7(1):45–73.

36. Constantino JN, Gruber CP. Social responsiveness scale (SRS-2). Torrance (CA): Western Psychological Services; 2012.

37. Gresham FM, Elliott SN. The social skills rating system. Circle Pines (MN): American Guidance Service; 1990.

38. Wolstencroft J, Robinson L, Srinivasan R, et al. A systematic review of group social skills interventions, and meta-analysis of outcomes, for children with high functioning ASD. J Autism Dev Disord 2018;48(7):2293–307.

39. Wong C, Odom SL, Hume KA, et al. Evidence-based practices for children, youth, and young adults with autism spectrum disorder: a comprehensive review. J Autism Dev Disord 2015;45(7):1951–66.

40. Reichow B, Volkmar FR. Social skills interventions for individuals with autism: evaluation for evidence-based practices within a best evidence synthesis framework. J Autism Dev Disord 2010;40(2):149–66.

41. Schreibman L, Dawson G, Stahmer AC, et al. Naturalistic developmental behavioral interventions: empirically validated treatments for autism spectrum disorder. J Autism Dev Disord 2015;45(8):2411–28.

42. Kroeger KA, Schultz JR, Newsom C. A comparison of two group-delivered social skills programs for young children with autism. J Autism Dev Disord 2007;37(5):808–17.

43. Kamps D, Thiemann-Bourque K, Heitzman-Powell, et al. A comprehensive peer network intervention to improve social communication of children with autism spectrum disorders: a randomized trial in kindergarten and first grade. J Autism Dev Disord 2015;45(6):1809–24.

44. Ichikawa K, Takahashi Y, Ando M, et al. TEACCH-based group social skills training for children with high-functioning autism: a pilot randomized controlled trial. Biopsychosoc Med 2013;7(1):14.

45. Solomon M, Goodlin-Jones BL, Anders TF. A social adjustment enhancement intervention for high functioning autism, Asperger's syndrome, and pervasive developmental disorder NOS. J Autism Dev Disord 2004;34(6):649–68.

46. Frankel F, Myatt R, Sugar C, et al. A randomized controlled study of parent-assisted children's friendship training with children having autism spectrum disorders. J Autism Dev Disord 2010;40(7):827–42.

47. Begeer S, Gevers C, Clifford P, et al. Theory of mind training in children with autism: a randomized controlled trial. J Autism Dev Disord 2011;41(8):997–1006.

48. Begeer S, Howlin P, Hoddenbach E, et al. Effects and moderators of a short theory of mind intervention for children with autism spectrum disorder: a randomized controlled trial. Autism Res 2015;8(6):738–48.

49. Thomeer ML, Lopata C, Volker MA, et al. Randomized clinical trial replication of a psychosocial treatment for children with high-functioning autism spectrum disorders. Psychol Sch 2012;49(10):942–54.

50. Rodgers JD, Thomeer ML, Lopata C, et al. RCT of a psychosocial treatment for children with high-functioning ASD: supplemental analyses of treatment effects on facial emotion encoding. J Dev Phys Disabil 2015;27(2):207–21.

51. Lopata C, Thomeer ML, Volker MA, et al. RCT of a manualized social treatment for high-functioning autism spectrum disorders. J Autism Dev Disord 2010;40(11):1297–310.

52. Laugeson EA, Frankel F. Social skills for teenagers with developmental and autism spectrum disorders: the PEERS treatment manual. New York: Routledge; 2011.

53. Laugeson EA, Frankel F, Mogil C, et al. Parent-assisted social skills training to improve friendships in teens with autism spectrum disorders. J Autism Dev Disord 2009;39(4):596–606.

54. Laugeson EA, Frankel F, Gantman A, et al. Evidence-based social skills training for adolescents with autism spectrum disorders: the UCLA PEERS program. J Autism Dev Disord 2012;42(6):1025–36.

55. Yoo HJ, Bahn G, Cho IH, et al. A randomized controlled trial of the Korean version of the PEERS® parent-assisted social skills training program for teens with ASD. Autism Res 2014;7(1):145–61.

56. Shum KKM, Cho WK, Lam LMO, et al. Learning how to make friends for Chinese adolescents with autism spectrum disorder: a randomized controlled trial of the Hong Kong Chinese version of the PEERS® intervention. J Autism Dev Disord 2019;49(2):527–41.

57. Rabin SJ, Israel-Yaacov S, Laugeson EA, et al. A randomized controlled trial evaluating the Hebrew adaptation of the PEERS® intervention: behavioral and questionnaire-based outcomes. Autism Res 2018;11(8):1187–200.

58. Schiltz HK, McVey AJ, Dolan BK, et al. Changes in depressive symptoms among adolescents with ASD completing the PEERS® social skills intervention. J Autism Dev Disord 2018;48(3):834–43.

59. Schohl KA, Van Hecke AV, Carson AM, et al. A replication and extension of the PEERS intervention: examining effects on social skills and social anxiety in adolescents with autism spectrum disorders. J Autism Dev Disord 2014;44(3):532–45.

60. Karst JS, Van Hecke AV, Carson AM, et al. Parent and family outcomes of PEERS: a social skills intervention for adolescents with autism spectrum disorder. J Autism Dev Disord 2015;45(3):752–65.

61. McVey AJ, Schiltz H, Haendel A, et al. Brief report: does gender matter in intervention for ASD? Examining the impact of the PEERS® social skills intervention on social behavior among females with ASD. J Autism Dev Disord 2017;47(7):2282–9.

62. Hong JK, Oh M, Bong G, et al. Age as a moderator of social skills intervention response among Korean adolescents with autism spectrum disorder. J Autism Dev Disord 2019;49(4):1626–37.

63. White SW, Ollendick T, Albano AM, et al. Randomized controlled trial: multimodal anxiety and social skill intervention for adolescents with autism spectrum disorder. J Autism Dev Disord 2013;43(2):382–94.

64. Walton KM, Ingersoll BR. Improving social skills in adolescents and adults with autism and severe to profound intellectual disability: a review of the literature. J Autism Dev Disord 2013;43(3):594–615.

65. Plavnick JB, Sam AM, Hume K, et al. Effects of video-based group instruction for adolescents with autism spectrum disorder. Except Child 2013;80(1):67–83.
66. Plavnick JB, Kaid T, MacFarland MC. Effects of a school-based social skills training program for adolescents with autism spectrum disorder and intellectual disability. J Autism Dev Disord 2015;45(9):2674–90.
67. Laugeson EA. PEERS® for young adults: social skills training for adults with autism spectrum disorder and other social challenges. New York: Routledge; 2017.
68. Gantman A, Kapp SK, Orenski K, et al. Social skills training for young adults with high-functioning autism spectrum disorders: a randomized controlled pilot study. J Autism Dev Disord 2012;42(6):1094–103.
69. McVey AJ, Dolan BK, Willar KS, et al. A replication and extension of the PEERS® for young adults social skills intervention: examining effects on social skills and social anxiety in young adults with autism spectrum disorder. J Autism Dev Disord 2016;46(12):3739–54.
70. Oswald TM, Winder-Patel B, Ruder S, et al. A pilot randomized controlled trial of the ACCESS program: a group intervention to improve social, adaptive functioning, stress coping, and self-determination outcomes in young adults with autism spectrum disorder. J Autism Dev Disord 2018;48(5):1742–60.
71. Morgan L, Leatzow A, Clark S, et al. Interview skills for adults with autism spectrum disorder: a pilot randomized controlled trial. J Autism Dev Disord 2014; 44(9):2290–300.
72. Smith MJ, Ginger EJ, Wright K, et al. Virtual reality job interview training in adults with autism spectrum disorder. J Autism Dev Disord 2014;44(10):2450–63.
73. Smith MJ, Fleming MF, Wright MA, et al. Brief report: vocational outcomes for young adults with autism spectrum disorders at six months after virtual reality job interview training. J Autism Dev Disord 2015;45(10):3364–9.
74. Krasny L, Williams BJ, Provencal S, et al. Social skills interventions for the autism spectrum: essential ingredients and a model curriculum. Child Adolesc Psychiatr Clin N Am 2003;12(1):107–22.
75. Park MN, Ellingsen R, Laugeson EA. Cognitive and behavioral interventions to improve social skills. In: Goldstein S, DeVries M, editors. Handbook of DSM-5 disorders in children and adolescents. Cham (Switzerland): Springer International Publishing; 2017. p. 637–50.
76. Laugeson EA, Park MN. Using a CBT approach to teach social skills to adolescents with autism spectrum disorder and other social challenges: the PEERS® method. J Ration Emot Cogn Behav Ther 2014;32(1):84–97.
77. Virués-Ortega J. Applied behavior analytic intervention for autism in early childhood: meta-analysis, meta-regression and dose-response meta-analysis of multiple outcomes. Clin Psychol Rev 2010;30(4):387–99.
78. Ashman R, Banks K, Philip RC, et al. A pilot randomised controlled trial of a group based social skills intervention for adults with autism spectrum disorder. Res Autism Spectr Disord 2017;43:67–75.
79. Hillier AJ, Fish T, Siegel JH, et al. Social and vocational skills training reduces self-reported anxiety and depression among young adults on the autism spectrum. J Dev Phys Disabil 2011;23(3):267–76.

Competitive Integrated Employment for Youth and Adults with Autism
Findings from a Scoping Review

Carol Schall, PhD[a],*, Paul Wehman, PhD[a,b], Lauren Avellone, PhD[a],
Joshua P. Taylor, MEd[a]

KEYWORDS

- Autism • ASD • Competitive integrated employment • Supported employment
- Customized employment

KEY POINTS

- The transition-to-work internship program called Project SEARCH plus ASD Supports (PS + ASD) had the highest level of research evidence.
- Supported employment was backed by substantial research as an evidenced-based practice for individuals with ASD.
- Specific components of vocational rehabilitation and transition program services (eg, community integrated service delivery, work experience before graduation) produced competitive employment outcomes for individuals with ASD.
- Technology supports in the workplace and customized employment emerged as promising practices with demonstrated efficacy across limited trials.
- Sheltered workshops were not identified as a means to competitive employment by this review and is thus not a recommended practice.

INTRODUCTION

Individuals with autism spectrum disorder (ASD) face significantly greater challenges transitioning to adult life than peers without disabilities and peers with other types of disabilities.[1] Research suggests that many individuals with ASD experience poor outcomes after leaving high school across a broad range of

[a] Department of Counseling and Special Education, Rehabilitation Research and Training Center, Autism Center for Excellence, School of Education, Virginia Commonwealth University, 1314 West Main Street, Box 842011, Richmond, VA 23284-2011, USA; [b] Department of Physical Medicine and Rehabilitation, Rehabilitation Research and Training Center, School of Medicine, Autism Center for Excellence, Virginia Commonwealth University, 1314 West Main Street, Box 842011, Richmond, VA 23284-2011, USA
* Corresponding author.
E-mail address: cmschall@vcu.edu

Child Adolesc Psychiatric Clin N Am 29 (2020) 373–397
https://doi.org/10.1016/j.chc.2019.12.001
1056-4993/20/© 2019 Elsevier Inc. All rights reserved.
childpsych.theclinics.com

Abbreviations	
ASD	autism spectrum disorder
CE	customized employment
CIE	competitive integrated employment
IDD	intellectual and developmental disabilities
IPS	individualized placement and support
PS + ASD	Project SEARCH plus ASD Supports
SE	supported employment
VR-JIT	virtual reality job interview training

life domains.[2] In addition, adolescents and young adults with ASD have higher incidences of anxiety and depressive disorders compared with peers without disabilities or other disabilities.[3] A heightened risk of anxiety and depression, combined with a greater likelihood of unsatisfactory postsecondary outcomes in major life areas highlights the vulnerability of individuals with ASD.[4] However, the current knowledge base concerning effective interventions for youth and adults with ASD is extremely limited.

Employment is the defining activity of adulthood and acts as a protective factor in the acquisition of many key life domains.[5] People with disabilities report that work is a source of identity, inclusion, financial support, and socialization.[6] Even so, securing competitive integrated employment (CIE) remains a primary challenge for many young adults with ASD. Although federal legislation has mandated enhanced services for transition, many young adults with ASD still face unemployment on leaving secondary education settings.[7,8] Findings from the 2017 National Autism Indicators Report showed that only 14% achieved paid work in an integrated setting, while the majority (54%) worked without pay usually in segregated settings.[9] Furthermore, 27% of adults with ASD reported no participation in work or other integrated community activities.[9] A review of employment outcomes for 47,312 individuals with ASD indicated an overall employment rate of only 37.57%.[10] Overwhelmingly, evidence highlights the tremendous need to improve employment outcomes for youth with ASD. The purpose of this scoping review was to identify key research describing effective employment interventions and practices for individuals with ASD seeking CIE.

METHOD

The following databases were reviewed to capture a broad range of multidisciplinary literature across educational, medical, and vocational rehabilitation related fields: PubMed, CINAHL, Education Research Complete, Web of Science, and EMBASE. The recommended framework for conducting a scoping review was followed, which includes formulating research questions, identifying relevant articles, and then charting and summarizing findings.[11–13] A more elaborate description of each step in the protocol is presented below.

Research Questions

The following research questions were developed to determine the range, nature, and extent to which evidenced-based employment practices for youth and adults with ASD have been investigated within the existing body of literature during the past 20 years:

- Which employment practices emerge at the highest levels of methodological rigor as effective interventions for individuals with ASD?
- What are the components of the interventions that appear to increase the employment outcomes for individuals with ASD?

Identification of Articles

The above-stated research questions led to the following inclusion criteria for published research studies:

1. Published between 2000 and 2019
2. Population samples where 100% of individuals had ASD with or without a comorbid diagnosis
3. Research examined interventions or practices resulting in CIE outcomes
4. Published in peer reviewed journals in the United States or abroad written in or translated into English

Articles were excluded if:

1. They did not meet criteria for methodological rigor as level I, experimental, level II, quasi-experimental, or level III, secondary data analysis research
2. The study did not examine CIE as an outcome of the intervention

Articles were reviewed by 2 researchers who met 95% inter-rater agreement in applying inclusion and exclusion criteria during the review process. Both researchers had previous training in research methodology and applicable disciplines related to the intersection of ASD and CIE. Key search terms used for study selection are presented in **Table 1**. A record of the total number of articles included and excluded at each stage is presented in **Fig. 1**.

Charting Findings

Articles collected during the review were categorized according to established guidelines ranking methodology and assigned an associated I–III ranking outlined in **Table 2**.[14] This scoping review restricted analysis to the top 3 levels of rigor to identify the most empirically based findings related to CIE interventions for individuals with ASD. All articles meeting inclusion criteria were subjected to 3 tiers of review: (1) screening for duplicates, (2) abstracts screened for inclusion/exclusion criteria, and (3) full text articles assessed for inclusion/exclusion criteria.

Table 1 Key search terms		
Format	**Population**	**Intervention**
Concept terms related to the main topic, organization of terms using Boolean operations (AND/OR/NOT), and truncation symbols by population × intervention	Autis* OR autism spectrum disorder OR asperger* OR ASD OR high functioning autis*	Evidence-based employment practice OR vocational rehabilitation OR employment practices OR supported employment OR customized employment OR competitive integrated employment OR employment internships OR transition to employment OR open employment

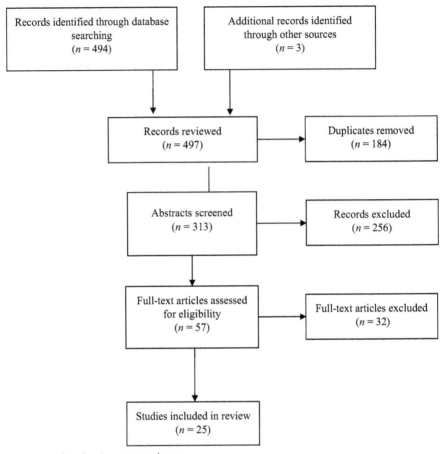

Fig. 1. Article selection process by stage.

RESULTS

A total of 25 articles met established inclusion criteria regarding employment interventions for individuals with ASD. Nearly all studies were conducted within the United States (n = 23; 92%), followed by the United Kingdom (n = 1; 4%), and Ireland (n = 1; 4%). A breakdown of articles by methodological rigor includes 6 at level I, 4 at level II, and 15 at level III.

Review of Level I Research and Findings

Level I is the highest level of methodological rigor using randomized control designs.[14] Of the studies identified at level I, the following findings emerged: (1) Project SEARCH plus ASD Supports (PS + ASD) is an effective transition-to-work program for youth and young adults with ASD and significant support needs; and (2) technology, such as virtual reality interviewing and a personal digital assistant (PDA), promotes job attainment and independence, respectively, in a vocational setting.[4,15–19] Each is reviewed in more detail.

PS + ASD Supports model

A total of 4 studies examined PS + ASD Supports, which is an extension of the traditional Project SEARCH model.[4,15–17] For context, the traditional model was developed in the

Table 2			
Research methodology rigor coding system			
Methodology	**Rank**	**Description**	**Types**
Experimental	I	• Random assignment to groups • Manipulation of independent variable • Tests of causality • Control of confounding variables	Randomized control designs, classic experimental designs that include randomization
Quasi-experimental	II	• Assignment is *not* random but all other experimental qualifications are met	Classic experimental designs that do *not* include randomization, preposttest designs, posttest only designs, interrupted time series designs
Non-experimental (Secondary Data Analysis)	III	• Assignment is not random • No control of extraneous variables • No causality. Relationship between variables examined	Correlational studies, predictive designs, model testing designs, regression analyses

Data from Newhouse R, Dearholt S, Poe S, et al. The Johns Hopkins Nursing Evidence-Based Practice Rating Scale. 2005. Baltimore, MD: The Johns Hopkins Hospital; Johns Hopkins University School of Nursing.

mid-1990s to help high school students with disabilities aged 18 to 22 years build work skills by participating in a series of individualized unpaid internships in applied business settings using supported employment (SE) techniques (**Table 3**).[20] Several key elements define the Project SEARCH model, including complete immersion in a workplace, personalized curriculums, customized internships, highly trained staff, collaboration among service provider agencies, braided funding streams, follow-along services, and a business-led approach.[20] Because Project SEARCH adheres to the principles of SE (see **Table 3**), it also focuses on securing CIE outcomes for all students after leaving the internship program regardless of the severity of disability.[15] In fact, Project SEARCH is designed for individuals with intellectual and developmental disabilities (IDD).

The PS + ASD Supports model follows the traditional Project SEARCH format but further includes the installation of diagnosis-specific supports that address the vocational, learning, social, and communication needs of individuals with ASD and IDD or other comorbid disorders. Results from our review suggested an extremely high rate of transition-to-employment using the PS + ASD model, with CIE outcomes ranging from 73.4% to 90% for participants with ASD and IDD, compared with a range of 6% to 17% employment for control groups.[15] Wehman and colleagues[4] attribute such noteworthy employment outcomes to several key components of the PS + ASD model, including the high dosage and intensity of the internships, use of evidenced-based teaching strategies known to be specifically effective for individuals with ASD, increased opportunities to conduct vocational assessments, applied opportunities for interns to build resumes before transitioning to work, a focus on collaboration with adult agencies, and a perpetually high work standard for interns. A more in-depth description of the key PS + ASD components that contribute to its success are presented in **Table 4**.

Table 3
Principles of supported employment

Component	Description
Presumption of employment	Anyone with a desire to work, can work, regardless of severity of disability.
Integrated employment	Individuals with disabilities should work in competitive, integrated jobs within the community.
Comparable wages	Individuals with disabilities should earn commensurate wages and benefits as those without disabilities performing similar work.
Self-determination	The individual with the disability should have control over guiding the job search process.
Focus on strengths	Individuals with disabilities are viewed in terms of abilities rather than deficits.
Power of supports	Focus is placed on identifying and installing vocational supports that will promote independence in the workplace.
Systems change	The SE approach recognizes the need for traditional systems that do not foster CIE outcomes to be changed.

Adapted from Wehman P, Revell WG, Brooke V. Competitive Employment: Has it become the "first choice" yet? J Disabil Policy Stud 2003;14(3):163-173; with permission.

Technology for employment skills

The remaining 2 studies identified at level I rigor highlighted the potential for technology to bolster CIE outcomes. Both of these studies were completed with more cognitively able individuals.[18,19] First, Gentry and colleagues[19] found that the use of an iPod touch as a PDA helped individuals with ASD and significant support needs

Table 4
Key components for success of the PS + ASD Supports model

Component	Description
Internships	Students are immersed in a work setting for over 700 h of internship experience. Internships are customized to meet individual student's strengths, needs, interests, and preferences.
Instructional strategies	Evidenced-based teaching strategies, such as applied behavior analysis, are used to teach vocational, social, academic, and communication skills.
Vocational assessment practices	Opportunities to asses skills and needs in applied settings are maximized due to the extensive amount of time spent in the work setting.
Resume/work history	Students leave the program with a developed resume, references, contacts, and applied skills developed in a work setting which bolster employability.
Seamless transition to adult services	Students begin working with adult service provider agencies immediately on entering the PS + ASD program so supports are installed long before they graduate.
Meeting business needs	Internships are real jobs that fill a real need within the business so students learn to meet high expectations for work standards.

organize employment tasks. Participants were taught how to use various applications on the device to meet job support needs, such as using tasks lists, picture prompts, task reminders, navigation tools, and task-sequencing prompts. Findings suggested that individuals taught to use the PDA required a significantly lower number of job support hours during the first 12 weeks of employment compared with control participants. Furthermore, this trend continued during a subsequent 12-week period.

Secondly, Smith and colleagues[18] used a Virtual Reality Job Interview Training (VR-JIT) program to help youth and young adults with ASD practice interviewing in a simulated environment. Data collected at a 6-month follow-up suggested that participants who received the VR-JIT training were more likely than control participants to have secured a competitive position within the community. However, it should be noted that results were collapsed in terms of types of position with competitive employment and volunteering reported as the same outcome. Volunteering along with any other type of nonpaid work is generally not considered an acceptable work outcome regardless of the level of community integration. Although both of these studies support the use of technology in teaching workplace independence, it is noted that only 2 studies were identified at level I methodology and thus more research in this area is needed to better understand the breadth of application.

Review of Level II Research and Findings

All 4 studies identified at level II rigor shared a common theme of an SE approach (see **Table 3**). SE is a packaged intervention that involves 4 phases; assessment phase (job seeker profile), supported job searching (job development), on-the-job training (job site training), and follow-along services (long-term supports). Individuals with ASD have disability-specific supports at each phase that appear to be unique to them.[21,22] For example, individuals with ASD have difficulty identifying their job preferences during the job seeker profile stage, usually because of a lack of employment experiences. In addition, they may require alternate interviewing strategies and a higher intensity of instruction to achieve independence at work during the job development and job site training phases.[21] Because of its personalization for each job seeker, SE provides an opportunity for those modifications without compromising fidelity of implementation.

Each article defined a set of intervention services that were individualized and adhered to an "employ then train" philosophy, which is a hallmark of SE. The SE approach refutes the need for preparatory training before immersion in a work setting and instead focuses on assisting an individual with a disability in finding employment and then adding needed supports to build skills and promote independence. Findings from articles identified at level II support the efficacy of the SE approach across both youth and adults with ASD.

For example, Wehman and colleagues[23] reported an 82% employment rate for participants using personalized SE with all participants earning at or above minimum wage and securing equal benefits to those without disabilities performing similar work. Most individuals in this study were described as having high social interaction support needs (76%) and partial to full travel support needs (84%), indicating that these individuals had significant support needs.[23] In a pilot study using the Individualized Placement and Support (IPS) model, which is an SE model that includes specialized supports for individuals with psychiatric disorders, McLaren and colleagues[24] reported that all 5 participants (100%) with ASD and a comorbid psychiatric condition were able to secure CIE positions in the community. These 5 individuals represented a mix of those with some college experience or college degrees (3) and those who acquired specialized certificates on graduation from high school (2). Similarly, Howlin and colleagues[25] reported a 68% employment rate for adults with "high functioning" (without comorbid IDD) ASD in 13 different industries using services that characterize the SE model, including job searching and workplace support. Lynas reported a 56% employment rate for adults with ASD across the range of cognitive abilities using Project ABLE in Ireland which defines itself as a "place, then train" SE model by providing customized services, such as job assessment, development of a job profile, and on-the-job supports.[26] Lynas noted that, in this case, all CIE outcomes were observed among the adult rather than the youth population involved with Project ABLE. Nevertheless, overall, the level II research findings provide strong support for the use of SE as an evidence-based intervention for individuals with ASD.

Review of Level III Research and Findings

There were 15 studies meeting criteria for level III research rigor. They used secondary data analysis to describe correlations between services delivered and CIE outcomes. Most focused on the correlation between specific VR services and CIE outcomes (n = 9).[10,27–34] Four studies examined the correlation between agency-specific services (eg, individuals with ASD who accessed SE services from a provider, individuals with ASD who accessed sheltered workshop services before CIE).[22,23,35,36] Two studies examined the correlation between transition services during high school and CIE outcomes after high school.[37,38] One study compared the correlation between 2 groups, one that received SE after PS + ASD during high school and one that received SE after graduation from high school (**Table 5**).[21] As these were secondary data analysis studies, most of these did not provide thorough reports of the cognitive abilities of those included in the research populations. These studies explored the correlation between 5 service delivery types and CIE outcomes. The services included: (1) VR, (2) SE, (3) customized employment (CE), (4) high school transition programs, and (5) sheltered workshop participation. Each of these is presented below.

Correlation between vocational rehabilitation services and competitive integrated employment outcomes

Most of the level III research studies reviewed the correlation between specific VR services and CIE outcomes. **Table 6** presents a list and description of services offered by most State VR agencies. Findings from this research suggested that individuals with ASD were more likely to achieve CIE after the following indicators:

- Using more VR services was significantly correlated with better CIE outcomes[10,27,30,31]
- Clients who obtained CIE used 2 times as many services as those who did not[27]
- The following services were positively correlated with better CIE outcomes
  - Postsecondary education, occupational/vocational training, on-the-job training, job readiness training, job search assistance, for transition-aged youth[28,29]
  - Assessment, diagnostic and treatment services, counseling/job guidance, job search support, job placement assistance, on-the-job support, transportation services, across all age ranges[29–33]
- Assessment and vocational rehabilitation counseling and guidance without job-related services were not correlated with CIE outcomes[34]
- Despite better CIE outcomes from VR services, the range of individuals successfully employed was still underwhelming, ranging between 36% and 37%[27,28]

Table 5
Articles by level of methodological rigor

Article	Method	Population	Intervention	Outcomes	Country
Smith et al,[18] 2015	Level I: Randomized controlled trial (RCT)	Youth with ASD ages 18–31 y n = 26	Virtual reality interviewing	• At a 6-mo follow-up, participants who received the VR-JIT training were more likely than controls to obtain a competitive position (although not necessarily competitive employment as competitive volunteering was included in the outcome measures).	United States
Gentry et al,[19] 2015	Level I: RCT	Adults with ASD n = 50	Personal digital assistant	• Individuals who were trained to use the digital assistant required less job coaching hours during the first 12 wk of employment compared with control participants.	United States
Wehman et al,[15] 2017	Level I: RCT	Youth with ASD ages 18–21 y n = 49	Project SEARCH with ASD Supports	• CIE outcomes observed for 90% of participants within 3 mo of completing the intervention and 87% were still employed 12 mo later. Only 6% of	United States

(continued on next page)

Table 5
(continued)

Article	Method	Population	Intervention	Outcomes	Country
				control participants were employed at 3 mo postgraduation and 12% at a 12 mo follow-up. • All employed SEARCH graduates were hired at or above minimum US federal wage.	
Wehman et al,[16] 2014	Level I: RCT	Youth with ASD ages 18–21 y n = 40	Project SEARCH with ASD Supports	• CIE outcomes observed for 87.5% of SEARCH participants compared with only 6.25% of the control group who received transition services as usual.	United States
Wehman et al,[4] 2019	Level I: RCT	Individuals with ASD ages 18–21 y n = 156	Project SEARCH with ASD Supports	• CIE outcomes observed for 73.4% of SEARCH participants 1 year after completion compared with 17% of control participants who received transition services as usual. • Employed SEARCH graduates earned at or above US federal minimum wage. • Employed SEARCH participants worked an average of 20 h per week.	United States

Study	Design	Population	Intervention	Outcomes	Country
Whittenburg et al,[17] 2019	Level I: RCT	Adults with ASD (18–22 y) n = 14	Project SEARCH with ASD Supports for military-connected participants	• 83.3% (5 of 6) secured competitive employment positions following program completion compared with 0% of controls. • 4 of 5 positions secured were federal positions.	United States
Howlin et al,[25] 2005	Level II: Quasi-longitudinal/experimental	Adults (18–56 y) with autism or Asperger syndrome n = 114	National Autistic Society prospects (focus on work preparation, job searching, and workplace support)	• 68% of clients became employed. • Job secured in 13 industries with most in administration, office/clerical, or technical work.	United Kingdom
Lynas,[26] 2014	Level II: Quasi-experimental	Youth and adults with autism spectrum condition n = 72	Project ABLE (supported employment model)	• 56% of adult participants (18 y and older) ultimately achieved full or part-time employment. • The most common type of employment was retail (47%) followed by administration (24%).	Ireland

(continued on next page)

Table 5
(continued)

Article	Method	Population	Intervention	Outcomes	Country
McLaren et al,[24] 2017	Level II: Quasi-experimental	Young adults with ASD and a comorbid psychiatric disorder n = 5	Pilot: individual placement and support for ASD	• All 5 participants secured competitive employment jobs. • Wage and number of hours were higher for participants after completing the IPS model than achieved in prior jobs before participating in the IPS model.	United States
Wehman et al,[23] 2012	Level II: Quasi-experimental	Adults with ASD n = 33	Personalized supported employment services	• 82% of 33 participants achieved CIE. • Employment outcomes included an average of 22.5 h and a range of 8–40 h per week. • Participants all earned at or above US federal minimum wage. • All participants earned comparable benefits to nondisabled coworkers performing similar work for similar hours per week.	United States

Alverson & Yamamoto,[10] 2017	Level III: Secondary Data Analysis -RSA-911	Youth and adult VR clients with ASD n = 47,312	State VR services	• Case closure associated with greater number of VR services received. • Odds of becoming employed increased nearly 5-fold with each additional service.	United States
Alverson & Yamamoto,[27] 2017	Level III: Secondary Data Analysis-RSA-911	Youth and adult VR clients with ASD n = 49,623	State VR services	• More VR services associated with better CIE outcomes. • Clients obtaining CIE used 2 times as many services as those that did not obtain CIE. • Mean of 37% secured CIE (successful case closure) over 10 y.	United States
Brooke et al,[22] 2018	Level III: Secondary Data Analysis-Agency Records	Adults with ASD referred for employment services n = 139	Extended supported employment services	• 104 participants achieved CIE outcomes. • Job retention was 74.3% at 18 mo.	United States
Burgess & Cimera,[28] 2014	Level III: Secondary Data Analysis-RSA-911	Individuals under age 22 y with ASD and a VR case closure n = 34,501	State VR services	• 36% were successfully employed through VR services. • Transition-age students with ASD were more likely to be employed via VR services than the overall population of individuals using VR services.	United States

(continued on next page)

Table 5
(continued)

Article	Method	Population	Intervention	Outcomes	Country
Chen et al,[29] 2015	Level III: Secondary Data Analysis-RSA-911	Adults with ASD n = 5681	State VR services	• The following services positively predicted CIE for transition-age individuals; postsecondary education, occupational/vocational training, and on-the-job training. • The following services positively predicted CIE across all age groups; counseling/job guidance, job placement assistance, and on-the-job support. • However, most who obtained a job were underemployed.	United States
Chiang et al,[37] 2013	Level III: Secondary Data Analysis-NLTS2	Youth and young adults with ASD n = 830	Transition-to-employment supports through secondary school	• Career counseling during high school associated with higher likelihood of being employed after leaving high school.	United States

Cimera et al,[38] 2013	Level III: Secondary Data Analysis-RSA-911	Transition-age young adults with ASD n = 906	Two additional years of early (ie, age 14 y) transition services	• Young adults with autism who received an additional 2 y of early transition services (ie, starting at age 14 y) were significantly more likely to be employed than matched pairs in states who began transition services at age 16 y.	United States
Cimera et al,[35] 2012	Level III: Secondary Data Analysis-RSA-911	Adults with autism n = 430	Sheltered workshop participation	• Individuals who were in sheltered workshops before entering supported employment had no difference in the rate of employment but earned less in wages and received higher service costs than matched peers who were not in sheltered workshops.	United States
Ditchman et al,[30] 2018	Level III: Secondary Data Analysis-RSA-911	Youth and young adults (ages 16–24 y) with ASD n = 2219	State VR services	• Receiving a greater number of the following 6 services lead to better employment outcomes; assessments, counseling, job placement, on-the-job training, job search support, transportation services.	United States

(continued on next page)

Table 5
(continued)

Article	Method	Population	Intervention	Outcomes	Country
Kaya et al,[31] 2016	Level III: Secondary Data Analysis-RSA-911	Youth and young adults (ages 16–25 y) with ASD n = 4322	State VR services	• Use of the following services lead to an increased likelihood of CIE; on-the-job support, job placement services, rehabilitation technology, occupational/vocational training, job search assistance, vocational counseling and guidance, and job readiness training. • Higher levels of education and receiving a greater number of VR services was associated with CIE outcomes.	United States
Kaya et al,[32] 2018	Level III: Secondary Data Analysis-RSA-911	Young adults (ages 19–25 y) with ASD n = 3243	State VR services	• Better CIE outcomes associated with receipt of the following services; job placement, on-the-job support, on-the-job training, maintenance, information referral, and diagnostic and treatment services.	United States

Study	Level/Design	Population	Intervention	Findings	Country
Migliore et al,[33] 2012	Level III: Secondary Data Analysis-RSA-911	Youth and young adults (ages 16–26 y) with ASD n = 2913	State VR services	• Job placements services was the strongest predictor of CIE outcomes.	United States
Nye-Lengerman,[34] 2017	Level III: Secondary Data Analysis-RSA-911	Adults with ASD n = 15,679	State VR services	• Lower likelihood of CIE at case closure with use of administrative rather than community-based supports.	United States
Schall et al,[21] 2015	Level III: Secondary Data Analysis-Agency Records	Youth and young adults with ASD n = 45	SE with or without Project SEARCH plus ASD Supports	• Project SEARCH plus ASD Supports group required fewer intervention hours, earned more, and had higher job retention rates than those with ASD receiving SE without ASD-specific supports.	United States
Wehman et al,[39] 2016	Level III: Secondary Data Analysis-Agency Records	Youth and young adults with ASD (ages 19–59 y with mean age of 26 y) n = 64	SE services	• 98.4% (63 of 64) participants secured CIE positions using SE.	United States

Table 6	
Example state virtual reality services	
Service Category	**Description**
VR counseling	Guidance services promoting CIE outcomes, including counseling related to benefits, vocational goals, social issues, medical problems, and so forth.
Assessment activities	Evaluative activities designed to determine personal strengths, vocational interests, concerns related to employment and desired employment outcomes.
Diagnostic and treatment	Activities designed to determine beneficial therapies (eg, occupational or physical therapy), medications, or intervention needs related to employment.
College or university training	Support to aid with the pursuit of advanced training in a college, university, or technical school for degree, nondegree or certificate programs.
Job search assistance	Assistance with interviewing, locating jobs, and building resumes, and so forth.
Job development	Activities related to securing a proper job match, which include networking with businesses and evaluating potential businesses for fit.

Adapted from Kaya C, Chan F, Rumrill P, et al. Vocational rehabilitation services and competitive employment for transition-age youth with autism spectrum disorders. J Vocat Rehabil 2016;45(1):13-83; with permission.

- Despite better outcomes with VR services, most individuals with ASD who acquired CIE still reported being underemployed[29]

These findings suggest that individuals with ASD who access job-related services are more likely to achieve CIE than those who do not.

Correlation between supported employment and competitive integrated employment outcomes

CIE outcomes after SE ranged from 98.4% to 100%.[21,22,39] SE was also associated with strong employment retention with 1 study reporting 87.1% at 18 months after CIE acquisition.[22] These particular studies urge caution in generalizing results to other agencies because of the specific training employment specialists serving individuals with ASD received in these studies. Given the quasi-experimental and secondary data analysis studies finding positive CIE outcomes from SE, it is fair to conclude that SE is an evidence-based practice for individuals with ASD.

Correlation between customized employment and competitive integrated employment outcomes

Two of the studies presented noted that a major source of successful CIE outcomes for individuals with ASD was CE. CE matches the unique strengths, interests, and support needs of the job candidate with the identified demands of the employer.[22,39,40] To achieve CIE through CE, the employment service provider and job seeker undergo a 4-phase process involving (1) Discovery, (2) Customized Job Development, (3) Individualized On-the-Job Supports, and (4) Long-Term Supports.[39] Brooke and colleagues[22] found 63% of 126 jobs worked by 104 individuals with ASD across 18 months were customized. However, Wehman and colleagues[39] found similar results with 52 of 72 jobs (72.2%) being customized for a group of 64 adults with ASD seeking employment.

Results from these studies suggest that CE is a promising intervention requiring more prospective research.

Correlation between transition to adulthood programs during high school and competitive integrated employment outcomes

Three of the studies explored the correlation between transition practices while in high school and CIE outcomes after high school. These findings suggest the following high school practices and interventions have been associated with CIE after high school:

- Having a paid job during high school[37]
- Participating in intensive school-to-work programs, such as PS + ASD[21]
- Receiving career counseling[37]
- Receiving transition planning services[37]
- Starting transition at 14 years old instead of the federally mandated age of 16 years[28]

Furthermore, Schall and colleagues[21] found that youth who participated in PS + ASD in high school required fewer intervention hours to secure CIE, retained jobs longer, and had higher wages than the SE only group. These findings emphasize the importance of high school curriculum and activities in preparing youth with ASD for CIE.

Correlation between sheltered workshop programs and competitive integrated employment outcomes

One study reviewed the RSA 911 database to compare the CIE outcomes of individuals who moved from sheltered employment to CIE to those who moved directly into CIE without previous sheltered workshop experiences.[35] They examined differences in employment rate, hours worked, wages, and service costs. Their findings suggested no differences between the 2 groups with respect to the rate of employment and hours worked. However individuals with ASD without previous sheltered workshop experiences earned 32.4% more and cost 59.8% less in VR services than their matched peers who had previous sheltered workshop experiences. This study finds that sheltered workshops cost more in services and pay less in CIE wages with no advantages in employment outcomes or hours worked.

DISCUSSION

This scoping review analyzed the experimental, quasi-experimental, and secondary data analysis research literature to identify employment interventions that result in CIE for individuals with ASD. In addition, the authors provided a description of the intervention components that appear to increase positive CIE outcomes. **Table 7** presents these findings. The results suggest strong evidence for 1 packaged intervention, PS + ASD. In addition, there is strong evidence of the efficacy of SE for individuals with ASD given the multiple quasi-experimental and secondary data analysis articles presented. Both VR and transition-to-employment high school programs are recommended, particularly specific components of those interventions, such as career counseling and intensive job support services. Although there have been 2 randomized controlled trials on technology supports for teaching interviewing skills, and increasing independence at work, more research is needed to identify how best to integrate technology into the overall array of supports provided to individuals with ASD seeking CIE. The same is true of CE. It seems that CE is a promising practice that might result in better outcomes for individuals with ASD; however, more research and guidance regarding specific ASD Supports are needed to confirm these findings.

Table 7
Employment intervention components and levels of evidence

Intervention	Recommendation Based on Research	Support Needs of Individuals Included	Components of Intervention
PS + ASD	Strongly recommended	Significant support needs, including those with IDD	• Internships • Applied behavior analysis instructional strategies • Personalized vocational assessment practices • Gain resume/work history • Seamless transition to adult services • Meeting business needs
SE	Strongly recommended	Varied across the spectrum of cognitive abilities	• Job seeker profile • Job development • Job site training • Long-term supports
VR	Recommended	Not determined in studies	• Job placement • On-the-job support • On-the-job training • Maintenance • Information referral • Diagnostic and treatment services • Vocational training • Job search assistance • Job readiness training • Other VR-provided services not listed

High school transition services	Recommended	Varied across the spectrum of cognitive abilities	• Paid job before graduation • Participating in intensive school-to-work programs • Career counseling • Transition planning services • Early transition services (starting at 14 y) • Postsecondary education counseling • Self-advocacy training • Job readiness training
CE	Emerging as recommended	Significant support needs, including those with IDD	• Discovery • Job search planning • Customized job development and negotiation • On-the-job support • Postemployment support
Technology supports for work skills and schedules	Emerging as recommended	Varied across the spectrum of cognitive abilities	• Cognitive digital aids • Digital task analyses • Visual task prompts • Navigation tools • Task reminders • VR-JIT
Sheltered workshops	Not recommended	Varied across the spectrum of cognitive abilities	• Segregated noncompetitive work settings • Enclave-based work • Subminimum wage employment

Both technology and CE are promising practices that could increase CIE outcomes for individuals with ASD. Finally, given the lack of any advantages and the noted disadvantages, we cannot recommend sheltered workshops as a viable intervention to increase CIE outcomes.

There are commonalities across the components of the various evidence-based interventions. Specifically, the most effective interventions include personalized assessment, evidence-based on-the-job training strategies, intensive interventions using multiple strategies to meet the job seekers needs, diagnoses-specific supports that address the social communication needs of individuals with ASD at work, and intervention in real environments. These components appear to be keys to ensuring CIE outcomes for individuals with ASD.

Limitations

There are several limitations to note associated with both scoping reviews in general and with this particular review. Although scoping review protocol does not require a quality filter for article selection, authors opted to apply such a filter by screening for, and ranking, articles according to research methodology.[12] Although the quality filter strengthens the validity of findings by scrutinizing research designs, a meta-analysis of results more commonly performed with systematic reviews was not conducted. Rather, a descriptive analysis of findings was presented per scoping review design, which lacks the statistical backing that could be provided by a meta-analysis.[12] In addition, scoping reviews involve broad research questions, which inevitably yield broad findings. Therefore, the results of this review still offer more general information about the types of interventions and services that are effective for individuals with ASD rather than information about how to match specific interventions to the wide spectrum represented by individuals with ASD. This last point is particularly important with respect to the wide spectrum of abilities and impact noted in ASD and the lack of common terminology to describe individual support needs across the variety of domains where an individuals with ASD might require supports. Thus, we have described the level of support needs required by individuals studied in the various intervention recommendations in **Table 7**.

With respect to limitations specific to this review, it is possible that the inclusion of non-English articles may have informed other results. Similarly, all studies were conducted in western countries, mainly the United States, which could limit the generalizability of findings to non-Western cultures. Finally, it is possible that unpublished research exists on this topic that may have been conducted at levels I, II, or III. Sources were acquired from scientific databases to allow for ranking due to methodology and to ensure peer review, and thus gray literature on ASD and CIE outcomes was not systematically investigated during the article collection process.

Implications and Future Directions

Findings from this scoping review revealed 2 salient gaps within the existing literature. First, there remains a lack of research on interventions conducive to CIE for individuals with ASD at the level I rigor. The overwhelming majority of studies in this review were secondary data analysis, which highlights the need for more randomized control and quasi-experimental designs to be conducted to inform better intervention and service provision. Secondly, the existing research at levels I and II note a clear lack in the amount of variation of interventions being examined at the highest levels of methodological rigor. Although the results of this review clearly suggest that SE is an evidence based practice, there remains much room for other interventions, such as CE to be tested experimentally or quasi-experimentally.

Future research suggestions include an emphasis on more varied employment outcomes beyond employed versus unemployed following intervention and services. In particular, deeper investigations into the quality of outcomes (eg, job retention, wage, opportunities for upward mobility) associated with different types of interventions would be beneficial. Future research should also consider manipulating aspects of interventions to determine maximum efficacy, such as the dosage of intervention or services, or the training levels needed by service providers to effectively boost CIE outcomes. It would be extremely helpful for researchers to develop a common language to describe the cognitive abilities and support needs of the individuals for whom CIE interventions are found to be efficacious. This would likely increase the precision with which field-based practitioners could match intervention to individual. Finally, future research should examine the effect of demographic variables within randomized designs. For example, while PS + ASD was highly effective in helping transition-age students secure employment, a similar study with an older population or population from an extremely rural area has not been conducted at the randomized controlled trial level of research to determine its effectiveness with these populations. This scoping review allowed for clear gaps in the literature to be identified and holds the potential to influence future research directions.

SUMMARY

Individuals with ASD continue to experience extremely poor employment outcomes, often remaining chronically unemployed or only finding work in segregated settings.[9] The challenges that individuals with ASD face in their quest to attain CIE can be mitigated by the implementation of evidence-based interventions. Therefore, the identification of highly effective vocational interventions is greatly needed to help an array of stakeholders, including individuals with ASD, service providers, educators, and vested community members allocate time and funds most efficiently. Although there is still much research work to do to develop more interventions, it is encouraging to report growth in the development of research literature that has resulted in sound recommendations for practice.

DISCLOSURE

The authors have nothing to disclose. This study was funded by the Disability and Rehabilitation Research Project (DRRP) grant no. 90DP005103 from the National Institute on Disability, Independent Living, and Rehabilitation Research (NIDILRR), and by the Congressionally Directed Medical Research Programs (CDMRP) Autism Research Program grant no. W81XWH16-1-0707. No IRB approval was necessary. This project was nonhuman research.

REFERENCES

1. Shattuck PT, Wagner M, Narendorf S, et al. Post-high school service use among young adults with an autism spectrum disorder. Arch Pediatr Adolesc Med 2011; 165(2):141–6.
2. Burke MM, Waitz-Kudla SN, Rabideau C, et al. Pulling back the curtain: issues in conducting an intervention study with transition-aged youth with autism spectrum disorders and their families. Autism 2019;23(2):514–23.
3. Croen LA, Zerbo O, Qian Y, et al. The health status of adults on the autism spectrum. Autism 2019;19(7):814–23.

4. Wehman P, Schall C, McDonough J, et al. Competitive employment for transition-aged youth with significant impact from autism: a multi-site randomized clinical trial. J Autism Dev Disord 2019. https://doi.org/10.1007/s10803-019-03940-2.

5. Saunders SL, Nedlec B. What work means to people with a work disability: a scoping review. J Occup Rehabil 2014;24:100–1.

6. Kocman A, Weber G. Job satisfaction, quality of life, and work motivation in employees with intellectual and developmental disability: a systematic review. J Appl Res Intellect Disabil 2018;31(1):1–22.

7. Individuals with Disabilities Education Improvement Act. 2004, 20 U.S.C. § 1400.

8. Workforce Innovation and Opportunity Act. 2014, 29 U.S.C. § 2801.

9. Roux AM, Rast JE, Anderson KA, et al. National autism indicators report: developmental disability services and outcomes in adulthood. Philadelphia: 2017. Available at: https://drexel.edu/autismoutcomes/publications-and-reports/publications/National-Autism-Indicators-Report-Developmental-Disability-Services-and-Outcomes-in-Adulthood/. Accessed October 15, 2019.

10. Alverson CY, Yamamoto SH. Employment outcomes for individuals with autism spectrum disorders: a decade in the making. J Autism Dev Disord 2018;48: 151–62.

11. Arksey H, O'Malley L. Scoping studies: towards a methodological framework. Int J Soc Res Methodol 2005;8:19–32.

12. Armstrong R, Hall BJ, Doyle J, et al. Cochrane update. "Scoping the scope" of a Cochrane review. J Public Health (Oxf) 2011;33:147–50.

13. Pham MT, Rajic A, Grieg J, et al. A scoping review of scoping reviews: advancing the approach and enhancing consistency. Res Synth Methods 2014;5(4):371–85.

14. Newhouse R, Dearholt S, Poe S, et al. The Johns Hopkins Nursing evidence-based practice rating scale. Baltimore (MD): The Johns Hopkins Hospital, Johns Hopkins School of Nursing; 2005.

15. Wehman P, Schall CM, McDonough J, et al. Effects of an employer-based intervention on employment outcomes for youth with significant support needs due to autism. Autism 2017;21(3):276–90.

16. Wehman PH, Schall CM, McDonough J, et al. Competitive employment for youth with autism spectrum disorders: early results from a randomized clinical trial. J Autism Dev Disord 2014;44(3):487–500.

17. Whittenburg HN, Schall CM, Wehman P, et al. Helping high school-aged military dependents with autism gain employment through project SEARCH + ASD supports. Mil Med 2019;1–6. https://doi.org/10.1093/milmed/usz224.

18. Smith MJ, Fleming MF, Wright MA, et al. Brief report: vocational outcomes for young adults with autism spectrum disorders at six months after virtual reality job interview training. J Autism Dev Disord 2015;45(10):3364–9.

19. Gentry T, Kriner R, Sima A, et al. Reducing the need for personal supports among workers with autism using an iPod touch as an assistive technology: delayed randomized control trial. J Autism Dev Disord 2015;45(3):669–84.

20. Daston M, Riehle JE, Rutkowski S. High school transition that works. Baltimore (MD): Brookes Publishing; 2012.

21. Schall CM, Wehman P, Brooke V, et al. Employment interventions for individuals with ASD: the relative efficacy of supported employment with or without prior project SEARCH training. J Autism Dev Disord 2015;45(12):3990–4001.

22. Brooke V, Brooke AM, Schall C, et al. Employees with autism spectrum disorder achieving long-term employment success: a retrospective review of employment retention and intervention. Res Pract Pers Sev Disabil 2018;43(3):181–93.

23. Wehman P, Lau S, Molinelli A, et al. Supported employment for young adults with autism spectrum disorder: preliminary data. Res Pract Pers Sev Disabil 2012; 37(3):160–9.

24. McLaren J, Lichtenstein JD, Lynch D, et al. Individual placement and support for people with autism spectrum disorders: a pilot program. Adm Policy Ment Health 2017;44:365–73.

25. Howlin P, Alcock J, Burkin C. An 8 year follow-up of a specialist supported employment service for high-ability adults with autism or Asperger syndrome. Autism 2005;9(5):533–49.

26. Lynas L. Project ABLE (autism: building links to employment): a specialist employment service for young people and adults with an autism spectrum condition. J Vocat Rehabil 2014;41:13–21.

27. Alverson CY, Yamamoto SH. Employment outcomes of vocational rehabilitation clients with autism spectrum disorders. Career Dev Transit Except Individ 2017;48:151–62.

28. Burgess S, Cimera RE. Employment outcomes of transition-aged adults with autism spectrum disorders: a state of the states report. Am J Intellect Dev Disabil 2014;119:64–83.

29. Chen JL, Sung C, Pi S. Vocational rehabilitation service patterns and outcomes for individuals with autism of different ages. J Autism Dev Disord 2015;45:3015–29.

30. Ditchman NM, Miller JL, Easton AB. Vocational rehabilitation service patterns: an application of social network analysis to examine employment outcomes of transition-age individuals with autism. Rehabil Couns Bull 2018;61:143–53.

31. Kaya C, Chan F, Rumrill P, et al. Vocational rehabilitation services and competitive employment for transition-age youth with autism spectrum disorders. J Vocat Rehabil 2016;45(1):13–83.

32. Kaya C, Hanley-Maxwell C, Chan F, et al. Differential vocational rehabilitation service patterns and outcomes for transition-age youth with autism. J Appl Res Intellect Disabil 2018;31(5):862–72.

33. Migliore A, Timmons J, Butterworth J, et al. Predictors of employment and post-secondary education of youth with autism. Rehabil Couns Bull 2012;55:176–84.

34. Nye-Lengerman K. Vocational rehabilitation service usage and outcomes for individuals with autism spectrum disorder. Research in Autism Spectrum Disorders 2017;41-42:39–50.

35. Cimera RE, Wehman P, West M, et al. Do sheltered workshops enhance employment outcomes for adults with autism spectrum disorder? Autism 2012;16(1):87–94.

36. Mavranezouli I, Megnin-Viggars O, Cheema N, et al. The cost-effectiveness of supported employment for adults with autism in the United Kingdom. Autism 2014;18(8):975–84.

37. Chiang HM, Cheung YK, Li H, et al. Factors associated with participation in employment for high school leavers with autism. J Autism Dev Disord 2013; 43(8):1832–42.

38. Cimera RE, Burgess S, Wiley A. Does providing transition services early enable students with ASD to achieve better vocational outcomes as adults? Res Pract Pers Sev Disabil 2013;38:88–93.

39. Wehman P, Brooke V, Brooke AM, et al. Employment for adults with autism spectrum disorders: a retrospective review of a customized employment approach. Res Dev Disabil 2016;53-54:61–72.

40. Wehman P, Schall C, Taylor J, et al. Vocational interventions. In: Rieske RD, editor. Handbook of interdisciplinary treatments for autism spectrum disorders. Cham, Switzerland: Springer Nature; 2019. p. 355–74.

Transitioning from Adolescence to Adulthood with Autism Spectrum Disorder

An Overview of Planning and Legal Issues

Nanette Elster, JD, MPH*, Kayhan Parsi, JD, PhD

KEYWORDS

- Autism • Transition • Planning • Adolescence • Adulthood • Legal • Ethical

KEY POINTS

- Transition from adolescence to adulthood presents a variety of challenges to individuals with autism spectrum disorder (ASD).
- A variety of legal mechanisms exist to help support the interests and autonomy of individuals with ASD.
- Individuals with ASD who are transitioning will need a variety of supports (financial, housing, education, transportation, health care).
- A potential solution to improving transition to adulthood is supported decision-making.

INTRODUCTION

The transition to adulthood is complex. It is defined by many objective milestones, including going to college, obtaining employment, moving away from parents, and building a family.[1] Transition is also defined by subjective milestones, including being able to care for oneself, make important decisions, and manage one's finances.[1] Transition from adolescence to young adulthood is challenging for neurotypical individuals as well as individuals with autism spectrum disorders (ASD). However, for autistic individuals, this transition is even more complicated and poses a range of legal and ethical considerations. This article discusses how existing legal and social constructs may exacerbate rather than diminish barriers and access for autistic adults and identifies current and potential legal and policy solutions to reducing current systemic barriers.

Neiswanger Institute for Bioethics, Loyola University Chicago Stritch School of Medicine, 2160 South First Avenue, Maywood, IL 60153, USA
* Corresponding author.
E-mail address: nelster@luc.edu
Twitter: @kayhanparsi (K.P.)

Child Adolesc Psychiatric Clin N Am 29 (2020) 399–408
https://doi.org/10.1016/j.chc.2019.11.003
1056-4993/20/© 2019 Elsevier Inc. All rights reserved.

BACKGROUND

The transition from adolescence to young adulthood is challenging not only for individuals with ASD but also for their parents and caregivers. Parents report many obstacles and barriers in trying to get needed services for their children. For example, in 1 study "parents of individuals with ASD (20.83%) and CP [cerebral palsy] (18.18%) reported greater barriers in navigating the service delivery system compared to parents of adults with DS [Down syndrome] (10.87%)."[2]

The study goes on to report that

> [p]ost hoc tests revealed that parents of adults with CP and ASD had significantly greater future planning barriers with respect to a lack of information (0.46 and 0.48, respectively) compared with parents of adults with DS (0.17). Parents of adults with DS (vs ASD and CP) also reported significantly less future planning barriers with respect to financial barriers ($F = 6.15$, $P<.001$, partial $\eta^2 = 0.06$). Post hoc tests revealed parents of adults with ASD had significantly greater financial barriers (0.61) compared with parents of adults with DS (0.29).[2]

The literature is clear that compared with individuals with DS, parents of young adults with ASD face greater challenges when it comes to a variety of markers of adulthood. Many parents refer to this transition of their adolescent children into young adults as "falling off the cliff"; experts in transition planning refer to this as the services cliff.[3] This cliff metaphor powerfully reflects the new reality wherein services for which young adults with ASD were once entitled to now become services for which they are merely eligible.

OVERVIEW

This article considers several factors related to transition planning from adolescence to young adulthood for autistic individuals:

1. Legal mechanisms to protect the interests of autistic individuals
2. Capacity
3. Needed supports
   a. Financial
   b. Housing
   c. Education
   d. Transportation
   e. Health care, including mental health care and oral health care
4. Eligible support mechanisms
5. Shared decision making: A potential solution to improving transition to adulthood

CURRENT LEGAL CONSIDERATIONS IN TRANSITION PLANNING

Transition planning is very individualized. Physical, psychological, and intellectual abilities will all influence how to best support autistic individuals in moving toward adulthood. These same factors will be considered in determining who should make decisions and how. A range of legal mechanisms exist to support or control decision making for individuals with disabilities, including guardianship, conservatorship, power of attorney for health care, and power of attorney for finances. Many of these mechanisms have state-specific eligibility requirements; therefore, this article discusses the concepts generally.

Because capacity to make decisions may wax and wane or may exist for some decisions but not others, determining which legal mechanism or mechanisms are most appropriate can be challenging. Making such a determination, however, is necessary in moving forward with any transition plan. Some transition plans may involve more than 1 mechanism or may require a periodic readjustment regarding decision making because circumstances of the individual with ASD will change as will those of the decision maker or makers. What follows is a brief description of some of the most commonly used mechanisms for decision making for individuals who lack or have limited capacity to make decisions in one or more areas of activities of daily living (ADL).

Guardianship

Guardianship is a legal proceeding whereby a court grants an individual or individuals certain rights and authority with regard to another individual.[4] Guardianship is typically pursued when a person is of the age of majority but is unable to manage various aspects of their lives. (Guardianship of children also occurs, but discussion of this is beyond the scope of this article.) A court of law must deem that adult individual to be incompetent to enter into certain kinds of activities. Guardianship can have different levels of authority. Partial guardianship may grant an individual with certain rights and responsibilities. For instance, a partial guardian may be able to make financial and health care decisions for a person with ASD, but leave other decisions to him or her. Adolescents with ASD who are in transition should be included in the discussion as to whether a full, partial, or no guardianship situation is indicated. Part of this discussion will necessitate what if any ADLs the adolescent has trouble managing, and most importantly, what the person for whom guardianship is sought desires.[5] Kirby and colleagues[1] recommend that "youth are engaged throughout this process so that their perspectives about their own interests, abilities, and limitations are considered as well as situational characteristics that are appealing to them."

For individuals at majority age with ASD who also have an intellectual disability, most commonly other concerned parties (typically parents) seek out guardianship. Guardianship can be fraught with challenges, even when pursued with the best of intentions. An adult in guardianship relinquishes a great deal of legal rights. Parents (and other interested parties) who seek guardianship for a young adult with autism should give careful thought about the gravity of their decision. As one commentator has observed, "Adults in guardianships often have fewer rights than convicted felons, and the process is rarely reversible."[6] In addition, once a guardian is appointed, making changes to that relationship is very arduous, and again, requires court intervention.

Conservatorship

Conservatorship is a slightly different legal category compared with guardianship, depending on the jurisdiction. Conservatorship grants legal rights to an individual to control the financial affairs of another person.[4] Guardianship grants broader legal authority over another (although a limited or partial guardianship can be created that limits one's authority over another's legal affairs. In this case, conservatorship and guardianship would be synonymous). Conservatorship may be indicated in young adults with ASD who have challenges with regard to managing finances. Other mechanisms, such as power of attorney or representative payee, that is discussed later, may also be implemented to manage finances.

Differences between Guardianship and Conservatorship

Both guardians and conservators are appointed by a court. Such appointments are only made after an individual is determined, by a court, to lack legal capacity. In order for appointment of a guardian and/or conservator, a court must determine that the person for whom guardianship is sought cannot

- Meet essential requirements for physical health, safety, or self-care because the respondent is unable to receive and evaluate information or make or communicate decisions, even with appropriate supportive services, technological assistance, or supported decision making; and
- The respondent's identified needs cannot be met by a protective arrangement instead of guardianship or other less restrictive alternative.[7]

Although this is a "model law" and has not been enacted in every jurisdiction (the above language is from a Washington state statute), it provides a helpful reference point given that laws related to guardianship and conservatorship differ from state to state.

Conservatorship typically refers to decisional authority over the property of another. The National Conference of Commissioners on Uniform State Laws in the Uniform Guardianship, Conservatorship, and Other Protective Arrangements Act defines a conservator as "a person appointed by a court to make decisions with respect to the property or financial affairs of an individual subject to conservatorship."[4] A guardian has broader authority and is defined as "a person appointed by the court to make decisions with respect to the personal affairs of an individual."[4] Guardians can make decisions about health care, housing, and even personal associations. Ultimately, guardianship and conservatorship are formal legal proceedings that involve a court of law. They should be viewed as a "last resort" when other legal mechanisms prove to be inadequate in protecting the interests of an adult with ASD.[6]

Power of Attorney

Less formal legal mechanisms exist to help support young adults with ASD, including a power of attorney for health care and power of attorney for finances. For instance, the power of attorney for health care is a legal document whereby a principal grants an agent or proxy authority to make health care decisions for the principal (typically if the principal loses decision-making capacity). This kind of power of attorney is usually associated with older individuals who may eventually lose decision-making capacity and want to have a trusted individual (typically a family member) make critical health care decisions. This kind of authority to make health care decisions is typically triggered when the principal lacks decision-making capacity. However, a durable power of attorney for health care can be executed that grants an agent decision-making authority for health care decisions immediately. This kind of durable power of attorney for health care may be indicated in situations whereby a young adult with ASD needs greater support for health care decision making.[8]

The power of attorney for finance limits an agent's authority to financial decision making. Similar to the power of attorney for health care, this power of attorney can take effect immediately, allowing an agent to make financial decisions for the principal.[9] In either instance, the selection of a decision maker is often based on that individual's ability to make a decision that is one that the incapacitated person would have made if able to do so. This concept is known as substituted judgment. If the individual not only currently lacks capacity but has had limited or no capacity before the designation of the power of attorney, then decisions should be made that are in the best interests of the incapacitated individual. Both standards can pose challenges in practice. The substituted judgment standard presumes that a principal who had capacity but no longer possesses it has shared their views and preferences with their agent. The best interest standard, which is typically what is used with pediatric patients, is often interpreted as an objective standard. However, as anyone who is familiar with controversial pediatric cases can attest, not everyone subscribes to the same views regarding what is in a person's best interests.

Representative Payee

Another possible mechanism for managing financial concerns is the appointment of a representative payee. For example, if a person is receiving benefits under Social Security or Supplemental Security Income (SSI), the Social Security Administration can "appoint a suitable representative payee (payee) who manages the payments on behalf of the beneficiaries."[10] The designee is often a friend or family member but may also be an organization.[11]

Privacy Protections

An important consideration is assessing how and by whom decisions should be made for an adult with ASD, because considerations of privacy are critical. Certain legally mandated privacy protections exist for adults. Two areas of federal regulation that governs what information can be shared by whom and with whom are in the areas of health privacy and educational privacy. The Health Insurance Portability and Accountability Act (HIPAA) is the federal law that governs the privacy of personal health information.[11] The Family Educational Rights and Privacy Act (FERPA) is the federal law that protects access to educational information about a student.[12]

Both HIPAA and FERPA are necessary considerations because adults with ASD do not relinquish their privacy rights because of their autism or any related intellectual disability (absent a guardianship arrangement). Privacy protections for those older than 18 without a guardian or conservator can only be waived in writing by the individual.

NEEDED SUPPORTS

Like neurotypical young adults, adolescents with ASD who are transitioning to adulthood require several supports. These supports include but are not limited to the following:

1. Financial
2. Housing
3. Education
4. Transportation
5. Health care (including mental and oral)

Other supports might include a range of social supports, including engaging in recreational activities, dating, alcohol use, and social media use. Because young adults with ASD represent a variety of capabilities, the level of support provided must be tailored to the needs of each individual.[13]

Financial

Financial support may mean providing a personal finance course for someone with ASD who lacks an intellectual disability but has challenges with managing personal finances. Another young adult with ASD may require a trusted person (typically a parent) be the financial power of attorney for the individual. Given that some benefits are income dependent, having a basic understanding of finances can ensure that one continues to be eligible for those supports.

Housing

With regard to housing, many young adults with ASD live at home with parents. Others may live in group homes. The deinstitutionalization movement started in the early 1970s facilitated adults with intellectual disabilities to live in more intimate settings. This trend culminated in the late 1990s with the US Supreme Court Decision, Olmstead v L.C., 527 U.S. 581 (1999). The Court rendered its holding under the Americans with Disabilities Act (ADA) finding that "public entities must provide community-based services to persons with disabilities when (1) such services are appropriate; (2) the affected persons do not oppose community-based treatment; and (3) community-based services can be reasonably accommodated, taking into account the resources available to the public entity and the needs of others who are receiving disability services from the entity."[14] Although the holding was not specific to persons with ASD, it has influenced housing for those with ASD.

Recently, a new movement has emerged that has specifically examined this question of appropriate housing for young adults with ASD.[15] Some are arguing for more campuslike environments for individuals with ASD. Such settings could potentially offer more services and opportunities for cultural and recreational activities compared with traditional group home settings. This setting would allow for adults with ASD to become more integrated into their communities.

Education

Education also poses interesting challenges. Once an individual has aged out of the public education system (typically by the age 22), they no longer are entitled to educational services. They may be eligible for services and may receive some accommodations, but cannot be discriminated against in educational settings. The previous entitlement regimen, however, is gone. Essentially, this becomes a shift from the Individuals with Disabilities Act, which is an entitlement protection, to the ADA, which only requires reasonable accommodation.[16]

Young adults with ASD may opt for a variety of educational opportunities. For instance, some traditional colleges and universities have special curricula for students with ASD (National Louis University and Elmhurst College). Other schools are specifically geared toward individuals with ASD and other learning disabilities (Beacon College, Landmark College). Also, many community colleges offer students with ASD specialized courses and curricula. Not all of these options, however, will result in a traditional bachelor's or associate's degree. In addition, vocational opportunities may also exist.

Transportation

Transportation is one of the major markers for emerging adulthood. Many adolescents acquire a driver's license when they turn 16. Because of deficits in executive functioning, adolescents with ASD may either delay or never acquire a driver's license. Many will depend on family members or ride-sharing services. If they live in a major city with a well-developed transit system, they may be able to navigate the various transit and bus lines. Almost every community offers some kind of transportation assistance for individuals with disabilities. Mobility provides a certain level of freedom and independence for young people, impacting employment, access to health care, and social integration.[17]

Health Care

Health care poses special challenges for young adults with ASD. As pediatric patients, these individuals typically relied on their parents to make health care decisions. As young adults, they may no longer see a pediatrician and are relying on internists and other adult care professionals who may have much less training and experience treating individuals with ASD. Such care is also not as coordinated once a young adult with ASD moves from pediatric care to adult care. Importantly, many individuals with ASD can still make health care decisions for themselves (absent guardianship). A recent movement away from guardianship has been supported decision making (as discussed later). This kind of model allows an individual with ASD to make health care decisions with the support of another trusted person, as opposed to completely relinquishing their decision-making rights under a guardianship model.

ELIGIBLE SUPPORT MECHANISMS

Adults with ASD may be eligible for a range of supportive services through state, federal, and local sources. Some of the most common services are discussed later, but what follows is in no way exhaustive.

One source of support available to adults with ASD is SSI through Social Security. This program "pays benefits to disabled adults and children who have limited income and resources."[18] SSI is income dependent, and thus, if income increases, SSI financial benefits may be diminished. Other sources of support, however, may still be available, including Medicaid benefits to cover health care expenses. The income eligibility requirements can be an impediment, however, to pursuing satisfying employment and perpetuates payment of the legally sanctioned subminimum wage.

Medicaid is a key source of support for noninstitutional housing for individuals with ASD. Although Medicaid does provide federal funding, this funding is a match of state funding rather than an independent stream of funding by Home and Community-Based Service Waivers under Section 1915(c) of the Social Security Act is an example.[19] The Centers for Medicare and Medicaid Services offers incentives to encourage states to develop programs supporting provision of noninstitutional services (**Box 1**).

Because these are state and federal partnerships, the contours will differ from state to state and therefore are beyond the scope of this discussion. For a robust discussion of residential options under Medicaid, please see Cooper R, "Medicaid Residential Options for People with Autism and Other Developmental Disabilities."[20]

Achieving a Better Life Experience Accounts (ABLE)

Some have argued that the strict asset and income caps on SSI and Medicaid have "limited take-up and viability in assisting adults with ASD to become independent."[21]

Box 1
Home and community-based service waiver program basics

To qualify for a Home and Community-Based Service waiver, states must:

- Demonstrate that providing waiver services will not cost more than providing these services in an institution
- Ensure the protection of people's health and welfare
- Provide adequate and reasonable provider standards to meet the needs of the target population
- Ensure that services follow an individualized and person-centered plan of care

From Medicaid.gov. Home & Community-Based Services 1915(c). Available at: https://www.medicaid.gov/medicaid/hcbs/authorities/1915-c/index.html. Accessed Sept 30 2019.

One recent development that may counteract these earning thresholds is the creation of an Achieving a Better Life Experience (ABLE) Account. With the 2014 passage of the Achieving a Better Life Act (Public Law 113–295), "Contributions to the account, which can be made by any person (the account beneficiary, family and friends), must be made using post-taxed dollars and will not be tax deductible for purposes of federal taxes; however, some states may allow for state income tax deductions for contributions made to an ABLE account."[22] Although created through federal legislation, ABLE accounts are state specific and states are not required to offer such programs. ABLE accounts afford "many individuals with disabilities . . . the ability to save money to meet their own personalized needs while remaining qualified for benefits programs that are critical to maintaining their health and well-being."[23]

The ADA is another potential support; however, it provides no direct benefits but rather protects against discrimination in places of public accommodation, such as housing and employment based on one's disability (ADA, https://www.ada.gov/pubs/adastatute08.htm). The ADA may also require that "reasonable accommodations" are made to support the individual identified as having a disability. These reasonable accommodations can include such things as an adapted physical environment, an assistive communication device, a service animal, and so forth.

SHARED DECISION MAKING: A POTENTIAL SOLUTION TO IMPROVING TRANSITION TO ADULTHOOD

Currently, only 2 states, Delaware and Texas, legally recognize supported decision making. The underlying principle expressed in the Delaware statute is that "[a]ll adults should be able to live in the manner they wish and to accept or refuse support, assistance, or protection as long as they do not harm others and are capable of making decisions about those matters."[24] In Texas, the stated purpose of the supported decision-making statute is to "recognize a less restrictive substitute for guardianship for adults with disabilities who need assistance with decisions regarding daily living but who are not considered incapacitated persons for purposes of establishing a guardianship. . ."[25]

Many organizations, including the American Bar Association[26] and The Arc,[27] support this approach. In part, this approach to decision making has been favored because "guardianship creates tension between respect for patient autonomy and concern for patient competency. . ."[28]

Supported decision making, in conjunction with measures other than guardianship, is one way to respect the autonomy of the person with ASD. Respect for autonomy also gives the person a voice not only in his or her own care but more generally with respect to what is or is not helpful to others with ASD. Given that ASD is a spectrum and not generalizable, legal recognition of supported decision making is 1 way to promote social justice for persons with ASD.

In surveying these various issues, adolescents who are transitioning into young adulthood must be treated as individuals with their own set of values and preferences. The adage "if you've seen one person with autism, you've seen one person with autism" certainly applies. Some individuals with ASD may require full guardianship. Others may require a conservator. Others may only need supported decision making with a trusted third party (which may be a parent or other appropriate person). Moreover, in outlining the various needs, the authors wish to highlight that this population of young people with ASD is not monolithic. However, they often do share similar challenges and concerns.

SUMMARY

One of the most difficult aspects of transitioning to adulthood for those with ASD and their caretakers is the complex web of services and supports that were once coordinated and provided by external sources, such as schools and health care professionals. As these former sources of support become increasingly diffuse and uncoordinated with no clear path to ensuring that the financial, housing, emotional, social, and medical needs of the individual are met, the hope is that any potential legal issues can be appropriately addressed. The variety of mechanisms described here recognizes that once the transition is complete, the person for whom decisions are being made is an adult with all the rights that come with such status. Ultimately, any plan must ensure a balance between the autonomy of adults with ASD while still protecting their interests if necessary.

DISCLOSURE

The authors have nothing to disclose.

REFERENCES

1. Kirby AV, Schneider M, Diener M, et al. "Who is going to pay for the WiFi?" Exploring adulthood from the perspectives of autistic youth. Autism Adulthood 2018;1:37–43.
2. Lee CE, Burke MM, Arnold CK, et al. Comparing differences in support needs as perceived by parents of adult offspring with Down syndrome, autism spectrum disorder and cerebral palsy. J Appl Res Intellect Disabil 2019;32:194–205.
3. Roux AM, Shattuck PT, Rast JE, et al. National autism indicators report: transition into young adulthood. In: Drexel AJ, editor. Life course outcomes research program. Philadelphia: Autism Institute, Drexel University; 2015. p. p13.
4. National Conference of Commissioners on State Laws. Guardianship conservatorship and other protective arrangements acts. 2017. Available at: https://www.uniformlaws. org/viewdocument/final-act-no-comments-13?CommunityKey=2eba8654-8871-4905-ad38-aabbd573911c&tab=librarydocuments. Accessed September 30, 2019.
5. Bradley V, Hiersteiner D, St. John J, et al. What do NCI data reveal about the guardianship status of people with IDD? National core indicators data brief. 2019. Available at: https://www.nationalcoreindicators.org/upload/core-indicators/ NCI_GuardianshipBrief_April2019_Final.pdf. Accessed September 30, 2019.
6. Demer LL. The autism spectrum: human rights perspective. Pediatrics 2018;14: S369–72.
7. RCW 11.130.265. Basis for appointment of guardian for adult. 2019 c437 301. Available at: https://app.leg.wa.gov/RCW/default.aspx?cite=11.130.265. Accessed September 30, 2019.
8. Commission on Law and Aging. Giving someone a power of attorney for your healthcare. 2011. Available at: https://www.americanbar.org/content/dam/aba/administrative/ law_aging/2011_aging_hcdec_univhcpaform.pdf. Accessed September 30, 2019.
9. AARP. Financial power of attorney. AARP fin and legal 2010. Available at: https://www.aarp.org/caregiving/financial-legal/info-2017/financial-power-of-attorney.html. Accessed September 30, 2019.
10. Social Security Administration. When people need help managing their money: representative payee. Available at: https://www.ssa.gov/payee/. Accessed September 30, 2019.

11. U.S. Department of Health and Human Services. Your rights under HIPAA. Available at: https://www.hhs.gov/hipaa/for-individuals/guidance-materials-for-consumers/index.html. Accessed September 30, 2019.

12. U.S Department of Education. Family Educational Rights and Privacy Act. Available at: https://www2.ed.gov/policy/gen/guid/fpco/ferpa/index.html. Accessed September 30, 2019.

13. Autistic Self Advocacy Network, Family Network on Disability. Roadmap to transition: a handbook for youth transitioning to adulthood. 2016. Available at: http://autisticadvocacy.org/wp-content/uploads/2016/11/Roadmap-to-Transition-A-Handbook-for-Autistic-Youth-Transitioning-to-Adulthood.pdf. Accessed September 30, 2019.

14. Olmstead: community integration for everyone. United States Dept. of Justice Civil Rights Division. Available at: https://www.ada.gov/olmstead/olmstead_about.htm. Accessed September 30, 2019.

15. Lutz A. Who decides where autistic adults live? The Atlantic 2015. Available at: https://www.theatlantic.com/health/archive/2015/05/who-decides-where-autistic-adults-live/393455/. Accessed September 30, 2019.

16. Brown K. Accommodations and support services for students with autism spectrum disorders (ASD): a national survey of disability resource providers. J Postsecond Educ Disabil 2017;30(2):141–56.

17. Curry AE, Yerys BE, Huang P, et al. Longitudinal study of driver licensing rates among adolescents and young adults with autism spectrum disorder. Autism 2018;22:79–488.

18. Social Security Administration. Supplemental security income benefits. Available at: https://www.ssa.gov/benefits/ssi/. Accessed September 30, 2019.

19. Social Security Act. Available at: https://www.ssa.gov/OP_Home/ssact/title19/1915.htm. Accessed September 30, 2019.

20. Cooper R. Medicaid residential options for people with autism and other developmental disabilities. 2012. Available at: https://iacc.hhs.gov/meetings/iacc-meetings/2014/full-committee-meeting/january14/Medicaid_Residential_Options_for_People_with_Autism_and_other_Developmental_Disorders.pdf. Accessed September 30, 2019.

21. Friedman N, Warfield Erickson M, Parish SL. Transition to adulthood for individuals with autism spectrum disorder: current issues and future perspectives. Neuropsychiatry 2018;3:181–92.

22. National Resource Center. About ABLE accounts. Available at: https://www.ablenrc.org/what-is-able/what-are-able-acounts/. Accessed September 30, 2019.

23. McGee CT, Ferguson GA. A primer on ABLE accounts, vol. 52. Richmond (VA): University of Richmond Law; 2017. p. 149–80.

24. 16 Del. Code Ann. 9402 (A)(b)(1).

25. Texas Estates Code, Sec. 1357.003:2015.

26. ABA. ABA urges supported decision making as less-restrictive alternative to guardianship. Bifocal 2018;38:95–6. Available at: https://www.americanbar.org/groups/law_aging/publications/bifocal/vol_38/issue-6–august-2017-/aba-urges-supported-decision-making-as-less-restrictive-alternat/. Accessed September 30, 2019.

27. The Arc. Autonomy, decision-making supports, and guardianship. 2019. Available at: https://thearc.org/position-statements/autonomy-decision-making-supports-guardianship/. Accessed September 30, 2019.

28. Bates K, Nourie CE, Hanks C, et al. Legal options, challenges and insights in supporting young adults with disabilities. SGIM Forum 2013;36(6):13.

Intersection of Eating Disorders and the Female Profile of Autism

Claire M. Brown, Mark A. Stokes, PhD*

KEYWORDS

- Autism • Female • Eating disorders • Anorexia • Comorbidity

KEY POINTS

- The female profile of autism describes an experience and presentation of autism that is unique and different from male individuals. Assumptions about autism, and diagnostic tools often do not reflect these sex-based differences, leading to underdiagnosis and late diagnosis of autistic female individuals.
- There is a moderate degree of comorbidity between autism and eating disorders, particularly anorexia nervosa. Research indicates that up to 30% of patients with anorexia are autistic or display a high level of autistic traits. These rates may change as our understanding of the overlap between these conditions improves.
- Standard eating disorder treatment options and settings may need to be modified to better accommodate autistic female individuals. Autistic traits, such as rigid thinking, difficulty communicating thoughts and feelings, and sensory processing abnormalities can hinder traditional approaches to eating disorder treatment.
- There are still a number of unknowns that make understanding the intersection of eating disorder and the female profile of autism challenging. These include the impact of sensory processing abnormalities, intellectual disability, and whether the experience of autistic women who received a timely diagnosis differs from those with latent autism.

INTRODUCTION

An increasing body of literature has found substantial overlap between autism spectrum disorder (henceforth, autism) and eating disorders (EDs) in female individuals,[1–3] despite these being seemingly unrelated conditions. EDs are a collection of psychological conditions that are characterized by abnormal dieting, eating and purging behaviors, and disturbed body image.[4] EDs are typically female dominated, with the

Author Note: In accordance with community preferences, this article uses identity-first language to describe individuals with a diagnosis of autism, and traits related to autism (ie, autistic person; autistic traits).

Deakin University, School of Psychology, Faculty of Health, 221 Burwood Highway, Burwood, Victoria 3125, Australia
* Corresponding author.
E-mail address: mark.stokes@deakin.edu.au

Child Adolesc Psychiatric Clin N Am 29 (2020) 409–417
https://doi.org/10.1016/j.chc.2019.11.002
1056-4993/20/© 2019 Elsevier Inc. All rights reserved.

childpsych.theclinics.com

peak age of onset ranging between 16 and 20 years for various ED subtypes.[5] Autism, by contrast, is not a mental illness, but a complex neurodevelopmental condition that results in impairments in social communication, and a pattern of restricted interests and repetitive behaviors.[4] Autistic traits are present in the early developmental period, and it is frequently diagnosed in childhood.[6] Here, we present an exploration of the unique female profile of autism, comorbidity between autism and EDs, treatment approaches, and priority areas for future research.

FEMALE PROFILE OF AUTISM

Autism is estimated to occur in approximately 1 in every 59 children.[7] It is currently diagnosed at a male-to-female ratio of 3:1,[8] although female individuals are thought to be underrepresented.[9] The sex disparity in rate of occurrence has been partially attributed to genetic factors. The "female protective effect" proposes that girls and women require a higher etiologic load to exhibit autistic impairments to the same extent as male individuals, and that the aforementioned sex ratio may be a consequence of the female protective effect.[10,11] Male individuals are thought to require fewer familial risk factors to display autistic traits, although no causal or protective gene loci have been identified.[12,13]

Autism is a clinically heterogeneous condition, and this is particularly apparent when considering the varied presentation between male and female individuals.[14–16] Autistic girls and women are thought to experience and express their autism in unique and nuanced ways, that often do not reflect historical descriptions, or dominant ideas that have been largely informed by observations of autistic male individuals.[9,14] Autistic girls and women are less likely to display restricted interests, and engage in repetitive behaviors,[17] and some studies have shown that they are more likely to experience sensory processing abnormalities.[18] Autistic girls and women are also more likely to attempt to camouflage their autism.[19] Camouflaging is conceptualized as the active and effortful process of using learned social and communicative behaviors in an attempt to mask difficulties related to their autistic traits. Research indicates that more than 90% of autistic girls and women have attempted to camouflage their autism to fit in social situations.[19,20] Camouflaging, it should be noted, is a taxing process that may allow autistic female individuals to superficially pass in social situations, while simultaneously experiencing high levels of stress and anxiety.[18] Camouflaging has been identified as a precursor to the development of clinical mental health issues, and as a risk marker for suicidality.[20,21]

BARRIERS TO DETECTION AND DIAGNOSIS OF AUTISTIC FEMALE INDIVIDUALS

Autistic female individuals are routinely underdiagnosed. Autism can be reliably diagnosed in early childhood,[22] although autistic female individuals frequently reach adolescence or adulthood without a diagnosis, despite clinical intervention for other conditions.[18,23] Loomes and colleagues[8] report that there is a disproportionate risk that female individuals who meet the autism diagnostic criteria will not receive a clinical diagnosis, as key observers and professionals are likely influenced by gendered and stereotyped understandings of autism. This is shown to make them less likely to refer girls and women for an autism assessment, and more likely to attribute autistic traits to other causes.[11,24]

The development of diagnostic criteria and tools are also areas that have been impacted by gender bias, as they are often not specific or sensitive enough to detect the unique female profile of autism. Lai and colleagues[9] suggest that female autistic presentation often falls below the clinical cutoff point, which results in many autistic female individuals not receiving a diagnosis until much later in life. The development of gender-specific thresholds for diagnostic tools has been proposed as a way of reducing the incidence of missed female cases,[25] although this has not yet eventuated in a meaningful way.

Camouflaging, as previously discussed, is a further factor that has been identified as contributing to the underdiagnosis and late diagnosis of autistic girls and women. Although camouflaging techniques can be used to hide social confusion, it is proposed that they also have the intended or unintended consequence of allowing autistic female individuals to avoid detection and diagnosis.[26] Autistic girls and women are observed to be better adept at hiding their impairments than male individuals, and thus, are less easily identified.[18]

COMORBIDITY

When considering the intersection of autism and EDs, it is essential to acknowledge the barriers to effective detection and diagnosis of autism in girls and women, as they complicate the picture of comorbidity overall. Importantly, it has been found that ED populations often contain latent autistic girls and women who have not been diagnosed, or girls and women who are identified as autistic through their participation in research.[23] As such, the discussion of comorbidity is best understood at both a diagnostic and trait level.

Autism is overrepresented among female individuals with an ED, although research remains limited. A 2013 review found an average autism prevalence rate of approximately 23% in individuals with any type of ED, with data predominantly coming from 6 longitudinal, community-based Swedish studies.[1] At an individual study level, autism prevalence in ED populations is reported at rates of up to 30%,[27] with the vast majority of autism cases diagnosed in anorexia nervosa (AN) subtype using the Autism Diagnostic Observation Scale (ADOS-2).[28–31] The literature is further scarce when considering other ED subtypes. The authors are aware of only one investigation, the study by Vagni and colleagues,[23] in which clinical diagnoses of autism were made in ED subtypes other than AN. Vagni and colleagues[23] found that 33% of ED participants were classified as autistic using criteria of the Diagnostic and Statical Manual of Mental Disorders, Fifth Edition, with no significant differences observed among ED subtype (AN, bulimia nervosa, and binge eating disorder). It is worth noting, however, that this result may be influenced by methodological choices. Vagni and colleagues[23] used The Ritvo Autism Asperger Diagnostic Scale-Revised (RAADS-R), which has been reported to be highly sensitive to identifying autistic adults,[32] whereas other available studies relied on self-reported autism diagnoses,[33] or included small sample sizes for ED subtypes other than AN.[27,28] This is an area that requires further targeted investigation, as the preponderance of comorbidity with AN may be influenced by measurement and sampling biases.

Much of the literature to date has instead explored the presence of autistic traits in AN populations, as the cognitive profiles of girls and women with AN often resemble deficits that are characteristic of autism.[34] Such features include extreme attention to detail and an impaired ability to see "the bigger picture" (weak central coherence[33]), a lack of cognitive flexibility (poor set-shifting[34]), and decreased ability to infer independent mental states that are different from their own (poor theory of mind[35]). The similarities continue when examining the behavioral manifestation of both conditions. Autisticlike behaviors observed in girls and women with AN include social anhedonia, the presence of rigid attitudes and behaviors, a tendency toward perfectionism, and narrow interests focused on food and weight, which appear to resemble the restricted interests and repetitive behaviors that are characteristic of autism.[28,36–38] Trait-level research has typically used autism screening measures rather than gold-standard assessment tools, adding to the complexity of understanding the true rate of comorbidity.

Research considering ED rates among known autistic individuals is definitively lacking. Pooni and colleagues[34] included an autistic subset in their investigation; however, found no categorical diagnoses of EDs in either male or female individuals. The study, however, had an unusually high male-to-female ratio of 16:4, rendering it less sensitive to female ED diagnoses. Studies examining comorbidity at a trait level have found autistic participants to display significantly more ED symptoms than typically developing individuals, across both male and female individuals.[33,39] Courty and colleagues[33] included a small, male-dominated autistic sample, and found that autistic participants reported greater ED symptoms in all domains than typically developing controls. These results, however, included a high degree of standard error, indicating substantial differences within the sample, possibly because of gender.

TREATMENT APPROACHES

It is important to highlight the distinction between interventions for autism and EDs, as they serve vastly different purposes. Interventions for aspects of autism typically involve a range of therapeutic strategies aimed to reduce the functional impact of autistic traits on day-to-day life for the individual, and improve long-term outcomes. Autism, although behaviorally defined, has neurobiological underpinnings, that by their nature are central to the person, and therefore immutable.[40] Thus, the goal of appropriate autism interventions is not to eradicate autism from the individual, which can confer many valued qualities, but to reduce the debilitating impact associated with some autistic traits. By contrast, EDs, and specifically AN, has the highest mortality rate of any psychiatric condition.[41] Treatments for Eds, therefore, are aimed at disease recovery through restoring healthy body weight after starvation, and targeting socio-emotional factors that are believed to contribute to the maintenance of the disorder.[42]

The development of autism-specific ED treatment approaches is still in its infancy, although the presence of autistic traits appears to be associated with chronic AN, and poorer long-term outcomes.[33,43] As such, modifications to typical ED treatment programs are thought to be necessary.[44] In a recent study, Kinnaird and colleagues[44] reported that clinicians and autistic individuals alike felt it necessary to recognize the complexity of differentiating between behaviors that may be attributable to both autism and Eds; in particular, those related to communication challenges, rigidity of thinking, behavior patterns and routines, and difficulty identifying underlying thoughts and emotions.[44] They suggested that the socio-communicative challenges typical of autism may hinder traditional ED treatment approaches.

Specific treatment protocols are yet to be established, although results from the few studies available indicate that the role of other mental health conditions, such as depression, anxiety, and obsessive compulsive disorder, may be more salient than the presence of autism or autistic traits.[43,45] Significant differences are noted with a greater need for either intensive day patient services,[43] or longer inpatient treatment[45] among patients with high autistic traits, but both studies extrapolate that treatment augmentation may reflect increased emotional needs, rather than needs related to autism.

PRIORITY AREAS FOR RESEARCH AND CLINICAL PRACTICE
Differentiation and Construct Validity: What Are We Actually Measuring?

Patients with AN are reported to record higher scores on autism screening tools than healthy controls, specifically when in the acute phase of their illness,[2] although with some question around the origin of such traits.[27] Stewart and colleagues[43] and Mandy and Tachnturia[27] noted that when people with restrictive EDs are in a state of starvation, their social, emotional, and cognitive processes are diminished, resulting in social withdrawal, a reduction in communication skills, and restricted or repetitive behaviors. They suggest that these autisticlike traits that are frequently observed in AN may highlight an inability to accurately discriminate between the 2 conditions, and the phenomena may be better accounted for by the impact of starvation on the brain. It is currently unknown, however, if such autisticlike traits are apparent in nonclinical starved populations, although this line of enquiry may help to differentiate between starvation state and true autistic traits.

The only available meta-analysis examining autism and AN concluded that individuals with AN displayed more autistic traits than their typically developing peers, although overall, they did not reach the suggested clinical cutoff for the widely used autism screening measure (Autism Quotient [AQ]).[2,46] Thus, it is proposed that the high rates of autistic traits reported in AN may reflect a problem of construct validity, rather than comorbidity between the conditions.[47] It is worth noting, however, that sensitivity issues inherent in the AQ indicate that autistic traits displayed by girls and women are not always effectively measured by the AQ.[48]

Focus on Autistic Female Individuals

Although the vast majority of research has started with an ED population and explored latent autism and autistic traits, very little work has explored the experiences of previously identified autistic female individuals. For example, sensory processing abnormalities are nearly ubiquitous among autistic adults and children.[49,50] Hypersensitivity to particular food textures, tastes, smells, and/or appearance occur in close to 90% of autistic children,[51] and have been identified as predictors of food avoidance, and intentional restriction of foods.[52,53] It is currently unknown whether these feeding and eating issues precede clinically significant EDs in autistic female individuals, and what role sensory processing abnormalities play in the maintenance of EDs. Similarly, it is currently unknown if camouflaging and attempts to blend into friendship groups, or meet gendered societal expectations may influence eating and dieting behavior in autistic women. Or, whether camouflaging, which is known to contribute to severe mental health issues, such as depression, anxiety, and suicidality,[20] increases the vulnerability and susceptibility to developing an ED in autistic female individuals. The literature in this field would benefit from large-scale, targeted studies that seek to understand whether the experiences of autistic female individuals who received a timely autism diagnosis differ from those with latent autism and a primary diagnosis of an ED.

Intellectual Disability

Although distinct from autism, it is reported that approximately half of all autistic individuals have a comorbid intellectual disability.[54] It is reported that among autistic individuals with a comorbid intellectual disability, some EDs are more frequently observed, including pica, rumination, regurgitation, and food refusal. The studies included in Gravestock's[55] review did not differentiate between genders, and as such, it is currently unknown if, and how, the presence of intellectual disability impacts the intersection of autism and EDs in female individuals. Research does, however, indicate that many girls are initially identified for an autism assessment because of the presence of an intellectual disability,[56] presumably reducing the risk of unidentified autism or autistic traits during ED treatment.

CLINICAL IMPLICATIONS

In a clinical setting, female individuals who present with an ED, particularly AN, may benefit from being screened for comorbid autism. Simultaneously, those presenting for an autism assessment also should be evaluated for EDs and aberrant eating behaviors. To increase their visibility, female-centric screening and diagnostic instruments will be crucial for enabling accurate and timely diagnosis. These must be sensitive enough to identify the female profile of autism, as individuals may have camouflaged their symptoms to the extent that they are not detected unless that line of investigation is pursued directly.

SUMMARY AND FUTURE DIRECTIONS

Presently there is a modest, but increasing body of literature examining the overlap between autism and EDs in girls and women. Most of the literature has focused on AN, in which girls and women are shown to display elevated levels of autistic traits, and up to 30% diagnostic comorbidity between the conditions. What is lacking from the current body of knowledge, however, is a theoretic framework capable of explaining why EDs and not autism constitutes the primary diagnosis in so many female cases. Similarly, there remains a lack of research and understanding of the ramifications of EDs in autistic populations. Little is known about how female individuals with a primary diagnosis of autism experience an ED, as well as the possible differences in treatment and outcomes.

DECLARATION OF INTEREST

C.M. Brown declares that she has no conflict of interest. M.A. Stokes declares that he has no conflict of interest.

REFERENCES

1. Huke V, Turk J, Saeidi S, et al. Autism spectrum disorders in eating disorder populations: a systematic review. Eur Eat Disord Rev 2013;21(5):345–51.
2. Westwood H, Eisler I, Mandy W, et al. Using the autism-spectrum quotient to measure autistic traits in anorexia nervosa: a systematic review and meta-analysis. J Autism Dev Disord 2016;46(3):964–77.
3. Westwood H, Tchanturia K. Autism spectrum disorder in anorexia nervosa: an updated literature review. Curr Psychiatry Rep 2017;19(7):41.
4. American Psychiatric Association. Diagnostic and statistical manual of mental disorders (DSM-5®). Arlington (VA): American Psychiatric Pub; 2013.
5. Stice E, Marti CN, Rohde P. Prevalence, incidence, impairment, and course of the proposed DSM-5 eating disorder diagnoses in an 8-year prospective community study of young women. J Abnorm Psychol 2013;122(2):445.
6. Johnson CP, Myers SM. Identification and evaluation of children with autism spectrum disorders. Pediatrics 2007;120(5):1183–215.
7. Baio J, Wiggins L, Christensen DL, et al. Prevalence of autism spectrum disorder among children aged 8 years—autism and developmental disabilities monitoring network, 11 sites, United States, 2014. MMWR Surveill Summ 2018;67(6):1.
8. Loomes R, Hull L, Mandy WPL. What is the male-to-female ratio in autism spectrum disorder? A systematic review and meta-analysis. J Am Acad Child Adolesc Psychiatry 2017;56(6):466–74.

9. Lai MC, Lombardo MV, Auyeung B, et al. Sex/gender differences and autism: setting the scene for future research. J Am Acad Child Adolesc Psychiatry 2015;54(1):11–24.

10. Robinson EB, Lichtenstein P, Anckarsäter H, et al. Examining and interpreting the female protective effect against autistic behavior. Proc Natl Acad Sci U S A 2013; 110(13):5258–62.

11. Duvekot J, van der Ende J, Verhulst FC, et al. Factors influencing the probability of a diagnosis of autism spectrum disorder in girls versus boys. Autism 2017; 21(6):646–58.

12. Gockley J, Willsey AJ, Dong S, et al. The female protective effect in autism spectrum disorder is not mediated by a single genetic locus. Mol Autism 2015;6(1):25.

13. Werling DM, Geschwind DH. Sex differences in autism spectrum disorders. Curr Opin Neurol 2013;26(2):146.

14. Halladay AK, Bishop S, Constantino JN, et al. Sex and gender differences in autism spectrum disorder: summarizing evidence gaps and identifying emerging areas of priority. Mol Autism 2015;6(1):36.

15. Allely CS. Understanding and recognising the female phenotype of autism spectrum disorder and the "camouflage" hypothesis: a systematic PRISMA review. Advances in Autism 2019;5(1):14–37.

16. Lai MC, Baron-Cohen S, Buxbaum JD. Understanding autism in the light of sex/gender. Mol Autism 2015;6:24.

17. Sipes M, Matson JL, Worley JA, et al. Gender differences in symptoms of autism spectrum disorders in toddlers. Res Autism Spectr Disord 2011;5(4):1465–70.

18. Lai MC, Lombardo MV, Pasco G, et al, MRC AIMS Consortium. A behavioral comparison of male and female adults with high functioning autism spectrum conditions. PLoS One 2011;6(6):e20835.

19. Lai MC, Lombardo MV, Ruigrok AN, et al, MRC AIMS Consortium. Quantifying and exploring camouflaging in men and women with autism. Autism 2017; 21(6):690–702.

20. Cassidy S, Bradley L, Shaw R, et al. Risk markers for suicidality in autistic adults. Mol Autism 2018;9(1):42.

21. Bargiela S, Steward R, Mandy W. The experiences of late-diagnosed women with autism spectrum conditions: an investigation of the female autism phenotype. J Autism Dev Disord 2016;46(10):3281–94.

22. Barbaro J, Dissanayake C. Autism spectrum disorders in infancy and toddlerhood: a review of the evidence on early signs, early identification tools, and early diagnosis. J Dev Behav Pediatr 2009;30(5):447–59.

23. Vagni D, Moscone D, Travaglione S, et al. Using the Ritvo Autism Asperger Diagnostic Scale-Revised (RAADS-R) disentangle the heterogeneity of autistic traits in an Italian eating disorder population. Res Autism Spectr Disord 2016;32:143–55.

24. Young H, Oreve MJ, Speranza M. Clinical characteristics and problems diagnosing autism spectrum disorder in girls. Arch Pediatr 2018;25(6):399–403.

25. Constantino JN, Charman T. Gender bias, female resilience, and the sex ratio in autism. J Am Acad Child Adolesc Psychiatry 2012;51(8):756–8.

26. Head AM, McGillivray JA, Stokes MA. Gender differences in emotionality and sociability in children with autism spectrum disorders. Mol Autism 2014;5(1):19.

27. Mandy W, Tchanturia K. Do women with eating disorders who have social and flexibility difficulties really have autism? A case series. Mol Autism 2015;6(1):6.

28. Wentz E, Lacey JH, Waller G, et al. Childhood onset neuropsychiatric disorders in adult eating disorder patients. Eur Child Adolesc Psychiatry 2005;14(8):431–7.

29. Rhind C, Bonfioli E, Hibbs R, et al. An examination of autism spectrum traits in adolescents with anorexia nervosa and their parents. Mol Autism 2014;5(1):56.

30. Westwood H, Mandy W, Tchanturia K. Clinical evaluation of autistic symptoms in women with anorexia nervosa. Mol Autism 2017;8(1):12.

31. Westwood H, Mandy W, Simic M, et al. Assessing ASD in adolescent females with anorexia nervosa using clinical and developmental measures: a preliminary investigation. J Abnorm Child Psychol 2018;46(1):183–92.

32. Ritvo RA, Ritvo ER, Guthrie D, et al. The Ritvo Autism Asperger Diagnostic Scale-Revised (RAADS-R): a scale to assist the diagnosis of autism spectrum disorder in adults: an international validation study. J Autism Dev Disord 2011;41(8):1076–89.

33. Courty A, Maria AS, Lalanne C, et al. Levels of autistic traits in anorexia nervosa: a comparative psychometric study. BMC Psychiatry 2013;13(1):222.

34. Pooni J, Ninteman A, Bryant-Waugh R, et al. Investigating autism spectrum disorder and autistic traits in early onset eating disorder. Int J Eat Disord 2012;45(4):583–91.

35. Huke V, Turk J, Saeidi S, et al. The clinical implications of high levels of autism spectrum disorder features in anorexia nervosa: a pilot study. Eur Eat Disord Rev 2014;22(2):116–21.

36. Baron-Cohen S, Jaffa T, Davies S, et al. Do girls with anorexia nervosa have elevated autistic traits? Mol Autism 2013;4(1):24.

37. Tchanturia K, Davies H, Harrison A, et al. Altered social hedonic processing in eating disorders. Int J Eat Disord 2012;45(8):962–9.

38. Oldershaw A, Hambrook D, Stahl D, et al. The socio-emotional processing stream in anorexia nervosa. Neurosci Biobehav Rev 2011;35(3):970–88.

39. Kalyva E. Comparison of eating attitudes between adolescent girls with and without Asperger syndrome: daughters' and mothers' reports. J Autism Dev Disord 2009;39(3):480–6.

40. Bölte S. Is autism curable? Dev Med Child Neurol 2014;56(10):927–31.

41. Smink FR, Van Hoeken D, Hoek HW. Epidemiology of eating disorders: incidence, prevalence and mortality rates. Curr Psychiatry Rep 2012;14(4):406–14.

42. Treasure J, Schmidt U. The cognitive-interpersonal maintenance model of anorexia nervosa revisited: a summary of the evidence for cognitive, socio-emotional and interpersonal predisposing and perpetuating factors. J Eat Disord 2013;1(1):13.

43. Stewart CS, McEwen FS, Konstantellou A, et al. Impact of ASD traits on treatment outcomes of eating disorders in girls. Eur Eat Disord Rev 2017;25(2):123–8.

44. Kinnaird E, Norton C, Stewart C, et al. Same behaviours, different reasons: what do patients with co-occurring anorexia and autism want from treatment? Int Rev Psychiatry 2019;31(4):308–17.

45. Tchanturia K, Adamson J, Leppanen J, et al. Characteristics of autism spectrum disorder in anorexia nervosa: a naturalistic study in an inpatient treatment programme. Autism 2019;23(1):123–30.

46. Baron-Cohen S, Wheelwright S, Skinner R, et al. The autism-spectrum quotient (AQ): evidence from Asperger syndrome/high-functioning autism, males and females, scientists and mathematicians. J Autism Dev Disord 2001;31(1):5–17.

47. Hiller R, Pellicano L. Anorexia and autism: a cautionary note. Psychologist 2013,;26(11):780.

48. Baron-Cohen S, Cassidy S, Auyeung B, et al. Attenuation of typical sex differences in 800 adults with autism vs. 3,900 controls. PLoS One 2014;9(7):e102251.

49. Tavassoli T, Hoekstra RA, Baron-Cohen S. The Sensory Perception Quotient (SPQ): development and validation of a new sensory questionnaire for adults with and without autism. Mol Autism 2014;5(1):29.
50. Ledford JR, Gast DL. Feeding problems in children with autism spectrum disorders: a review. Focus Autism Other Dev Disabl 2006;21(3):153–66.
51. Marshall J, Ware R, Ziviani J, et al. Efficacy of interventions to improve feeding difficulties in children with autism spectrum disorders: a systematic review and meta-analysis. Child Care Health Dev 2015;41(2):278–302.
52. Lane AE, Young RL, Baker AE, et al. Sensory processing subtypes in autism: association with adaptive behavior. J Autism Dev Disord 2010;40(1):112–22.
53. Hull L, Petrides KV, Allison C, et al. "Putting on my best normal": social camouflaging in adults with autism spectrum conditions. J Autism Dev Disord 2017; 47(8):2519–34.
54. Simonoff E, Pickles A, Charman T, et al. Psychiatric disorders in children with autism spectrum disorders: prevalence, comorbidity, and associated factors in a population-derived sample. J Am Acad Child Adolesc Psychiatry 2008;47(8): 921–9.
55. Gravestock S. Eating disorders in adults with intellectual disability. J Intellect Disabil Res 2000;44(6):625–37.
56. Dworzynski K, Ronald A, Bolton P, et al. How different are girls and boys above and below the diagnostic threshold for autism spectrum disorders? J Am Acad Child Adolesc Psychiatry 2012;51(8):788–97.

Obsessive–Compulsive Disorder in Autism Spectrum Disorder Across the Lifespan

Markian Pazuniak, MD[a], Scott R. Pekrul, MD[b],*

KEYWORDS

- Autism spectrum disorders (ASD) • Obsessive–compulsive disorder (OCD)
- Obsessions • Compulsions • Stereotypic behaviors • Restricted interests

KEY POINTS

- Obsessive–compulsive disorder and autism spectrum disorder have overlapping behaviors that can be difficult to differentiate.
- Key to distinguish repetitive behaviors primary to autism spectrum disorder from those unique to obsessive–compulsive disorder are: autism spectrum disorder-only the behaviors are calming, sensory seeking, and ego-syntonic, whereas in obsessive–compulsive disorder they are ego-dystonic, cause distress, and driven by anxiety.
- Diagnostic scales can be used including the Children's Yale-Brown Obsessive Compulsive Scale for ASD.
- Pharmacology studies have shown mixed results but we recommend starting with an selective serotonin reuptake inhibitor, being mindful of the increase risk for side effects with patients with autism spectrum disorder.
- Exposure-response prevention can be used with patients with obsessive–compulsive disorder and autism spectrum disorder but modifications are necessary.

Autism spectrum disorder (ASD) and obsessive–compulsive disorder (OCD) are both common pediatric psychiatric conditions with a prevalence of rate in recent studies of 1% to 2% and 1% to 3%, respectively.[1–3] OCD is characterized by intrusive thoughts, images, or urges (obsessions) with purposeful mental or physical actions (compulsions) aimed at reducing anxiety caused by the obsession.[4] ASD can be characterized as impairments in social relationships and social-emotional reciprocity, and nonverbal communication combined with restricted and repetitive actions and interests.[4] Before the publication of the *Diagnostic and Statistical Manual of Mental Disorders* IV-TR, the diagnostic criteria of ASD or OCD precluded the diagnosis of the other disorder.[5,6]

[a] Department of Child and Adolescent Psychiatry, University of Maryland Medical Center, 701 West Pratt Street, 2nd Floor, Baltimore, MD 21201, USA; [b] Sheppard Pratt Health System, 6501 North Charles Street, Baltimore, MD 21204, USA
* Corresponding author.
E-mail address: spekrul@sheppardpratt.org

Child Adolesc Psychiatric Clin N Am 29 (2020) 419–432
https://doi.org/10.1016/j.chc.2019.12.003
1056-4993/20/© 2019 Elsevier Inc. All rights reserved.

childpsych.theclinics.com

Abbreviations	
ASD	Autism spectrum disorder
ASD-OCD	ASD and comorbid OCD
ASD-only	ASD and without OCD
CYBOCS-ASD	Children's Yale-Brown Obsessive Compulsive Scale for ASD
OCD	Obsessive–compulsive disorder

These exclusionary criteria were in part based on the idea that repetitive, restricted behavior as well as narrow and fixated interests found in ASD seemed to be similar to the obsessions and compulsions found in OCD. However, research suggests differences exist in the repetitive and restricted behavior between the 2 disorders. Further, studies indicate children and adolescents with ASD and comorbid OCD (ASD-OCD) may have unique symptomatology compared with patients with ASD and without OCD (ASD-only). Given the differences in treatment approaches between ASD and OCD, it is import for the clinician to recognize the similarities and differences between the 2 disorders to guide the most effective therapeutic interventions. This article reviews prior literature regarding the prevalence, diagnosis, and treatment in children and adolescents with autism and comorbid OCD from a developmental perspective.

EPIDEMIOLOGY

Individuals at any age with ASD are 2 times more likely to be diagnosed with OCD than the general population[7] with a suggested a comorbidity rate of 6% to 37%.[8,9] Within the pediatric population, 1 meta-analysis published in 2011 suggests a prevalence rate of 12.5% or 17.4%m depending on the methodology used.[10] OCD symptoms were more prevalent in children with ASD than matched children diagnosed with an anxiety disorder and children with no psychiatric diagnosis.[11] Parents of children with ASD rated their children as having higher obsessive–compulsive symptoms than parents of children with other anxiety disorders.[11] Parent's report of obsessive and compulsive symptoms yielded a higher comorbidity rate (20.2%) than the frequency based on the child's report (10.7%).[12] However, a selection bias may occur because these comorbid rates might be reflective of how children with ASD-OCD have more severe symptoms, which leads to more referrals to psychiatric care.[8,13]

Children and adolescents diagnosed with OCD are at increased risk of being diagnosed with ASD. In addition, 4% to 8% of children and adolescents diagnosed with OCD are diagnosed with ASD.[14] A diagnosis of ASD is 4 times more likely to be present in a youth diagnosed with OCD.[7] A survey of an outpatient clinic sample placed the frequency rate of Autism in children with OCD at 3.8%.[15] Subthreshold symptoms of ASD were also found to be elevated in pediatric patients with OCD compared with controls, with ranges from 18% to 35%.[13,16–18] Tics, symptoms of attention deficit hyperactivity disorder, and pathologic doubt, but not patient's insight, were correlated with increased symptoms of ASD within the OCD population.[17]

FAMILY HISTORY

Family history suggests a common etiology between OCD and ASD. Increased family history of ASD and ASD symptoms in youth with OCD has been observed in a few studies. Higher OCD symptoms were found in mothers of children with ASD-only and increased ASD symptoms are found in mothers of children with OCD-only.[16] ASD-only youth with higher scores on the repetitive behavior domain of the ADI-R and on the narrow restricted interests and rituals domain of the ADI-R were more likely to have parents with higher scores on Yale-Brown Obsessive-Compulsive Scale checklist.[19] Youth who displayed more complex stereotypies and repetitive movements are also more likely to have relatives diagnosed with OCD compared with those who displayed simple stereotypies and repetitive movements.[19,20]

PRESENTATION OF SYMPTOMS

The diagnosis of OCD in a child with ASD can be challenging. The previous exclusion of comorbid OCD and ASD before *Diagnostic and Statistical Manual of Mental Disorders*-IV unfortunately limited additional research on this topic in the past.[5,6] One of the complications is that children with ASD and language impairment add to diagnostic challenges because these patients often have difficulty conveying their thoughts and internal states.[21] Further, many individuals with ASD struggle with emotion identification and decreased insight, which can impact their ability to self-report symptoms.[21] Conversely, OCD symptoms may mask an underlying ASD diagnosis, especially if the child is on the autism spectrum and higher functioning.[14,22] Therefore, obsessive and compulsive symptoms may have to be ascertained via behavioral observation to a greater extent in those with ASD than without ASD.

There are many complications differentiating compulsive behavior in OCD-only from restricted and repetitive movements in ASD-only. For example, restrictive and repetitive behaviors that are more complex in ASD-only often present as similar to obsessions and compulsions in OCD-only.[5,23] In contrast, a child with OCD-only can present with the same severity of rigid and repetitive behavior, which are both higher than typically developing youth.[24] For a diagnosis of OCD, the repetitive behavior has to be impairing, which is difficult to assess in children with ASD owing to the reasons discussed elsewhere in this article.[24] ASD-only youth who acted out their favorite television or book characters are more likely to endorse obsessive and compulsive symptoms than ASD-only youth who are simply fixated with an with a toy or object, or those who collect facts about a topic.[25]

Although restricted and fixed interests in ASD-only can seem to be similar to obsessions in OCD-only, several diagnostic factors can help the clinician to separate these 2 features. For example, patients with ASD-only are likely to view their obsession or restricted interest as a source of pleasure (ie, ego syntonic) or as an interest that is engaging. Conversely, patients with OCD-only are more likely to be disturbed by their obsessions (ie, ego dystonic).[24,26,27] Further, fixed interests and restricted and repetitive movements are a source of validation, anxiety relief, and security for individuals with ASD-only.[27] Individuals with OCD-only will make an effort to avoid thinking about the obsessions, which they view as unacceptable, intrusive, and a source of anxiety[28] However, children with ASD-only may not view the intrusive thoughts as harmful or distressing.[26]

Overall, youth (ages 7–16 years old) with OCD-only report a higher number of obsessions (except religious obsessions, which were similar between the 2 disorders) than youth with ASD-only.[24] A second study finds more mixed results with youth diagnosed with OCD-only exhibiting more aggressive obsessions than children with ASD-only.[29] In contrast, children with ASD-only are more likely to exhibit hoarding behaviors than OCD-only and the general population, but the difference between ASD-only and OCD-only did not reach statistical significance.[29] Hoarding has been reported to be a common obsession in children and adolescents with ASD.[25,29] It is important to note that these papers only diagnosed youth as either OCD-only or ASD-only, so none of these individuals were diagnosed as comorbid ASD-OCD.

OCD compulsions can seem to be similar to the restricted, repetitive behaviors and stereotypies of ASD. Similar to how obsessions and restricted interests can be distinguished via careful observations, compulsions can also be differentiated from restricted and repetitive behaviors. One key element of compulsions in OCD is that the act itself is disturbing and maladaptive, unlike the restricted and repetitive behaviors of ASD, which are pleasurable and ego-syntonic.[7,8,21,28,30] In fact, the behavior of restricted and repetitive behaviors in ASD may be a goal in themselves for the individual.[28] One case study discusses a child with ASD-OCD combined who had an elevated heart rate and irritable affect when unable to complete his compulsion.[31] Children with OCD-only reported an overall greater number of compulsions compared with children with ASD-only.[24] In ASD-only youth, higher rates of repetitive movements are related to a greater number of obsessions.[24] Additionally, compulsive symptoms, as measured via the Repetitive Behaviors Scale–Revised compulsive score subset, is slightly inversely proportional with IQ.[32]

Studies are inconclusive with respect to which type of compulsion is more common in ASD versus OCD.[24,29] Ordering type compulsions are more common in OCD-only compared with ASD-only in 1 study and checking compulsions are more common in OCD compared with ASD in a second study[24,29] For youth, the compulsions in ASD-only are less elaborate and complex than in OCD-only.[24] Several compulsions, including repeating (56%), ordering (21%–56%), hoarding (25%–28%), and other compulsive behaviors (41%) are more prevalent in ASD-only patients than OCD-only patients.[25,29,33] Some of these compulsions, such as ordering, are positively correlated with severity of restricted interests in children and adolescents with ASD-only.[25]

Within the adult population, hoarding is noted to be more common in both the OCD-only and ASD-only populations.[34] In comparison with adults with ASD-only, those with OCD-only are found to have more repeating compulsions, but similar amounts of cleaning, checking, counting, arranging, and hoarding compulsions.[35] Again, it is important to note that many of these studies investigating compulsions and repetitive behavior did not take into account a possible ASD-OCD combined group. Instead, the studies separated subjects into only their primary diagnosis. However, a few of the studies did create an ASD-OCD group, which they compared with youth with OCD-only or youth with ASD-only. In these studies, the ASD-OCD combined group were more likely to display restricted and repetitive behaviors and interests as well as sensory motor behaviors compared with the ASD-only group.[36] There were conflicting studies for whether the obsessions in ASD-OCD combined groups were less severe or more severe than in OCD-only youth.[11,37,38] The ASD-OCD combined group may be associated with a greater prevalence of religious obsessions and a lesser prevalence of checking and washing compulsions compared with the OCD-only group.[38] The prevalence of many compulsions (including touching, tapping, rubbing, or ordering) and the prevalence of many obsessions (sexual, aggressive, or contamination) were similar between the ASD-OCD combined group and the OCD-only group.[15,38] Hoarding was present in 34% of children and adolescents with ASD-OCD, with 7% exhibiting severe hoarding behavior.[39]

ASD-OCD children were found to have poor insight.[29] Children with OCD-ASD combined had fewer prosocial behaviors and more difficulty relating with peers compared with their peers with OCD-only.[15] Adults with ASD-OCD combined blamed themselves significantly less for their intrusive thoughts when compared with OCD-only patients. Further, patients with ASD-OCD combined believed significantly less that their thoughts can cause harm when compared with those with OCD-only.[26] ASD-OCD youth were also more likely to be diagnosed with social phobia, attention deficit hyperactivity disorder, and separation anxiety compared with their OCD-only counterparts.[38]

In adults with OCD-ASD combined, there is conflicting evidence as to whether obsessive and compulsive severity and presentation differed between the comorbid group, the OCD-only group, and the ASD-only group. In 1 study, compulsive symptoms were found to be more prevalent than those with ASD-only.[40] The compulsion types that were more common in adults with ASD-OCD included repeating, touching, tapping, hoarding, and ordering as well as sexual obsessions.[9,34,40] Cleaning, checking, counting, and aggressive obsessions and compulsions were less likely in the ASD-OCD group than in OCD-only group.[40] Hoarding was also common in the ASD-only group.[40]

DIAGNOSTIC TOOLS

Current diagnostic and rating scales developed for and used in OCD do not take into consideration the diagnosis of comorbid ASD.[21] However, some scales have been adopted to include an ASD diagnosis. For example, the Children's Yale-Brown Obsessive Compulsive Scale for ASD (CYBOCS-ASD) may be a reliable adaptation of the widely scale for obsessions and compulsions for comorbid OCD and ASD.[21] A scale such as the Obsessive Compulsive Inventory–Revised may also be helpful to separate restrictive and repetitive behaviors in ASD from compulsions primary to OCD.[23,40] The Kiddie Schedule for Affective Disorders and Schizophrenia has an adaptation for patients with Autism and includes questions to assess for OCD symptoms.[21] The Autism Co-morbidity Interview–Present and Lifetime Version was created to assess for co-morbid symptoms of anxiety with reliability and validity for OCD.[33] The Children's Inventory for Psychiatric Syndromes–Parent Version also has promise to assess for OCD in ASD.[21] Functional behavioral analysis may be helpful with the diagnosis of OCD in the ASD population, because it could uncover obsessions as possible antecedents for the targeted behavior, and compulsions or relief of prior anxiety as the consequence of the action.[41]

TREATMENT

Obsessive and compulsive symptoms in children and adolescents with comorbid ASD-OCD are more resistant to treatment than the OCD-only population.[22,42] General recommendations for treatment may require adapting existing treatments of OCD to address the unique challenges of those with ASD.

Both psychotherapy and psychopharmacology have some evidence to support their efficacy. Multiple studies, including a few randomized control studies, showed efficacy of cognitive behavioral therapy (CBT) in the combined OCD and ASD population.[43–47] A case study and 1 case series suggested that CBT may even be efficacious in individuals who have low functioning ASD or a severe cognitive disability.[31,48] Conversely, another study did not support CBT in this population because it did not separate from the anxiety management therapy, which functioned as the control.[47] Additionally, CBT was found to be less effective in the ASD-OCD group compared with the OCD-only group.[49] One limitation of these studies was that some may have focused mostly only on those who individuals with ASD who are considered higher functioning.[21] Another limitation was that 1 study only had 25% of the study population in the adolescent age range.[47] A lack of parent training for some of the CBT treatments was reported to be another limitation.[43]

Similar to their counterparts with ASD-only, children with ASD-OCD may also benefit from social skills training.[23] Social skills training and CBT can help youth with ASD-OCD in specific ways. For example, combining social skills training with CBT provides knowledge of what behaviors one can do in a specific situation, which is sometimes a difficulty for patients with comorbid ASD and OCD.[26]

Adaptations in the CBT protocol for OCD have been made to the comorbid ASD-OCD population.[46] The general CBT protocol for OCD consists of 5 components:

1. Psychoeducation
2. Fear hierarchy development
3. Exposure/response prevention
4. Cognitive strategies
5. Generalization/relapse prevention[43,50,51]

Prior studies indicate that CBT treatments were on average 17 sessions long with each session lasting between 35 minutes and 2 hours.[43] The decrease in compulsive behavior did not decrease until after the exposure response prevention plan was completed.[43] Adjustments that were made to CBT for this population account for the difficulty in completing thought diaries or considering alternate thinking strategies.[49] Young children with ASD may require more structured CBT therapy and cognitive restructuring may be less helpful.[23] Further modifications to the CBT program included more psychoeducation on affective identification and anxiety, creating a timeline for the sessions with the amount of time spent on each activity to create more structure, and identifying triggers for dysregulation. Additional adaptations found helpful included greater parental involvement, increasing a child's awareness of his or her compulsive behavior, use of preferred interests of the patient in the examples, increased use of visual aids, and positive reinforcement.[43,52,53] Exposure and relapse prevention are conducted at home rather than at the clinic in this case study for the findings to become generalizable with the exposure and response prevention tasks conducted by the parent at the end of each session.[53] Overall, less focus was placed on cognitive techniques in the OCD-ASD group than in an OCD-only group.

Evidence for the efficacy of psychopharmacologic treatment for comorbid ASD and OCD remains mixed and limited. Common complications of psychopharmacologic treatment was that those with ASD may be more sensitive to the activating side effects of a selective serotonin reuptake inhibitor.[21] Because risperidone and aripiprazole are approved for the treatment of irritability in ASD, they are both drugs that have been investigated for its possible role in OCD. Two studies show a marginal, but statistically significant, decrease in obsessions and compulsions with Aripiprazole use as measured by the CYBOCS-ASD (95% confidence intervals in 2 separate studies is a 0.27–1.77 decrease and a 1.65–4.35 decrease).[54,55] However, treatment with risperidone was not associated with an improvement in CYBOCS-ASD scores from placebo.[56] Additionally, a later 2016 Cochrane review combined the data of the 2 studies of aripiprazole and concluded that aripiprazole did not differentiate from placebo in reducing CYBOCS-ASD score (95% confidence interval of decrease, 3.86–0.00).[57] Within the adult population, risperidone was associated with a mild decrease in the CYBOCS-ASD score from 16.15 ± 3.58 to 12.77 ± 3.63 ($P<.01$), which separated from placebo[58,59]

Selective serotonin reuptake inhibitors are used as first-line psychopharmacologic treatment for the OCD-only population.[60,61] However, its effectiveness within the pediatric comorbid OCD and ASD population remains mixed. Citalopram was not found to separate from placebo in reducing CYBOCS-ASD scores.[62] For children and adolescents, fluoxetine, at low dosages (9.9 ± 4.35 mg), was associated with a decrease in repetitive behaviors, but not with an improvement in the Clinical Global Improvement scale.[63] However, the improvement in CYBOCS-ASD score was not replicated in a much larger study at a similar dosage.[64] Fluvoxamine is poorly tolerated in the ASD-OCD pediatric group. Only 1 of the 18 children randomized to fluvoxamine clinically improved in a 12-week double blind placebo-controlled study.[65] Fluvoxamine was found to reduce OCD symptoms in adults with ASD in a small study of 30 adults[66]

Clomipramine was associated with a decrease in the OCD symptoms for those with ASD-OCD combined, which separated from placebo.[67] Average dose of clomipramine in the study is 152 mg/d.[67] A case study suggests that deep brain stimulation of the nucleus accumbens in an adult patient with ASD, refractory OCD, and aggression may decrease OCD symptoms as measured from the CYBOCS-ASD with effects lasting for up to 1 year.[68]

PROGNOSIS

Increased autistic traits in children with OCD increased functional impairment, but was not associated with OCD severity.[18] However, this paper suggested that intensive family involvement may have acted as a mediating factor (Griffiths). Advancing age is correlated with fewer compulsive behaviors.[69] A comorbid diagnosis was not related to the severity of compulsions.[69] Many of the features associated with a poorer prognosis in ASD (difficulties in interpersonal relationship, hoarding, presence of a cluster A personality disorder) were also associated with poor outcomes in those with ASD-OCD.[22]

SUMMARY AND RECOMMENDATIONS

The diagnosis of comorbid OCD and ASD can be difficult to make because the symptomology of OCD and ASD can seem similar. Further, children and adults on the autism spectrum can present with a wide variation in terms of severity and those with language impairment who are lower functioning will have increased limitations in self-report. However, even those individuals on the autism spectrum who are considered higher functioning can often present with poor insight and have challenges conveying their internal states. It may therefore be more critical for the clinician to rely on observation and caregiver reports regardless of language delay. However, as reported, some OCD scales such as the CYBOCS-ASD have been modified for ASD and can be used clinically for diagnosis and monitoring progression of treatment. Identification of situations and mental states that precede episodes of emotional and behavioral dysregulation as well as behaviors associated with relief can also aid in the diagnosis of OCD in ASD. One of the key features that clinicians can use to distinguish repetitive behaviors primary to ASD from OCD-only is that in ASD-only the behaviors are often calming, sensory seeking, and ego-syntonic, whereas in OCD they are often ego-dystonic, cause distress, and are primarily driven by anxiety. Further, OCD symptoms may appear as new behaviors and different from baseline stereotypic behaviors the individuals with autism may have displayed for an extended periods of time before the onset of OCD. Hoarding in a child or adolescent with ASD may indicate a comorbid ASD-OCD diagnosis. The type of obsessions and compulsions in pediatric ASD-OCD may be similar to those with OCD-only, but some evidence suggests that there may be fewer checking and washing compulsions and more religious obsessions in the combined ASD-OCD group. More studies are recommended to discern which obsessions and compulsions are more common in the ASD population, because there have been conflicting studies with respect to diagnosis.

In regard to treatment, if a person on the autism spectrum has been diagnosed with OCD, we recommend following standard clinical guidelines for OCD with some modifications. For example, we recommend starting with a modified CBT for ASD for those that are deemed higher functioning and/or with good expressive-receptive language abilities. Specifically, exposure and relapse prevention can be helpful, especially with adaptations to fit children and adults with ASD. Such adaptations may include more structure, greater emphasis on affective identification, less emphasis on cognitive schema modulation, and home sessions to increase generalizability of therapy. Although studies have not shown reliable efficacy for a specific medication to treat OCD in patients with ASD, there is some evidence to support the use of clomipramine, fluoxetine, and fluvoxamine. Lower dosages of fluoxetine are found to be effective in a few studies. However, because persons with ASD tend to have higher rates of side effects with psychotropic medications, we recommend starting with a selective serotonin reuptake inhibitor that has evidence for efficacy in OCD-only and using the principle of start low and go slow.

Although we recommend starting with CBT and adding a medication if there is poor or only partial response, some on the autism spectrum, especially if they are lower functioning and/or have significant language delay, may be unable or unwilling to participate in therapy. For those individuals, it may be necessary to start with a psychotropic intervention in addition to standard behavioral interventions for ASD. If first-line treatment with a selective serotonin reuptake inhibitor is either ineffective or demonstrates only a partial response after 2 trials, it may be necessary to try clomipramine. If clomipramine is either not tolerated, ineffective, or shows a partial response, the clinician can consider augmenting or replacing these medications with a second-generation antipsychotic that has evidence for efficacy in OCD such as risperidone or aripiprazole.[70–98] However, it should be noted that there were mixed results when using risperidone and aripiprazole in comorbid ASD-OCD. An advantage of using either risperidone or aripiprazole is they have approval from the US Food and Drug Administration for irritability related to ASD in children.

Suggested topics for future research include (1) possibly identifying specific subgroups within the OCD-ASD group, because this patient population may be a heterogeneous grouping that can have different pathology, presentation, and treatment; (2) further elaborating adaptations in the CBT protocol for the different functional levels of ASD; (3) and additional randomized controlled trials that measure the efficacy of selective serotonin reuptake inhibitors and antipsychotics.

DISCLOSURE

The authors have nothing to disclose.

REFERENCES

1. Lai MC, Lombardo MV, Baron-Cohen S. Autism. Lancet 2013;383(9920):1–14.
2. Calas J, Hernandez-Martinez C, Cosi S, et al. The epidemiology of obsessive-compulsive disorder in Spanish Children. J Anxiety Disord 2012;26:746–52.
3. Rapoport JI, Inoff-Germain G, Greenwald MM, et al. Childhood Obsessive-compulsive disorder in the NIMH MECA Study: parent versus child identification of cases. J Anxiety Disord 2000;14:535–48.
4. American Psychiatric Association. Diagnostic and statistical manual of mental disorders. 5th edition. Arlington (VA): American Psychiatric Association; 2013.
5. Jiujias M, Kelley E, Hall L. Restricted, repetitive behaviors in autism spectrum disorder and obsessive-compulsive disorder: a comparative review. Child Psychiatry Hum Dev 2017;48:944–59.
6. American Psychiatric Association. Diagnostic and statistical manual of mental disorders, vol. IV-TR. Washington, DC: American Psychiatric Association; 2006.

7. Meier SM, Petersen L, Schendel DE, et al. Obsessive-Compulsive Disorder and autism spectrum disorders: longitudinal and offspring risk. PLoS One 2015;10: e0141703.
8. van der Plas E, Dupuis A, Arnold P, et al. Association of autism spectrum disorder with obsessive-compulsive and attention-deficit/hyperactivity traits and response inhibition in a community sample. J Autism Dev Disord 2016;46:3115–25.
9. Kerns CM, Kendall PC. The presentation and classification of anxiety in autism spectrum disorder. Clinical Psychol Sci Prac 2012;19:323–47.
10. Van Steensel FJ, Bögels SM, Perrin S. Anxiety disorder in children and adolescents with autistic spectrum disorders: a meta-analysis. Clin Child Fam Psychol Rev 2011;14:302–17.
11. Russell E, Sofronoff K. Anxiety and social worries in children with Asperger syndrome. Aust N Z J Psychiatry 2005;39:633–8.
12. Bitsika V, Sharpley C. Variation in the profile of anxiety disorders in boys with an ASD according to method and source of assessment. J Autism Dev Disord 2015; 45:1825–35.
13. Weidle B, Melin K, Drotz E, et al. Preschool and current autistic symptoms in children and adolescents with obsessive-compulsive disorder (OCD). J Obsessive Compuls Relat Disord 2012;1:168–74.
14. Arildskov TW, Hojgaard DR, Skarphendinsson G, et al. Subclinical autism spectrum symptoms in pediatric obsessive-compulsive disorder. Eur Child Adolesc Psychiatry 2016;25(7):711–23.
15. Mack H, Fullana MA, Russell AJ, et al. Obsessions and compulsions in children with Asperger's Syndrome or high-functioning Autism: a case-control study. Aust N Z J Psychiatry 2010;44:1082–8.
16. Ozyurt G, Besiroglu L. Autism spectrum symptoms in children and adolescents with obsessive compulsive disorder and their mothers. Noro Psikiyatr Ars 2018; 55:40–8.
17. Ivarsson T, Melin K. Autism Spectrum Traits in children and adolescents with obsessive-compulsive disorder (OCD). J Anxiety Disord 2008;22:969–78.
18. Griffiths DL, Farrell LJ, Waters AM, et al. ASD traits among youth with obsessive-compulsive disorder. Child Psychiatry Hum Dev 2017;48:911–21.
19. Hollander E, King A, Delaney K, et al. Obsessive compulsive behaviors in parents of multiplex autism families. Psychiatry Res 2003;117:11–6.
20. Abramson RK, Ravan SA, Wright HH, et al. The relationship between restrictive and repetitive behaviors in individuals with autism and obsessive compulsive symptoms in parents. Child Psychiatry Hum Dev 2005;36:155–65.
21. Postorino V, Kerns CM, Vivanti G, et al. Anxiety disorders and obsessive-compulsive disorder in individuals with autism spectrum disorder. Curr Psychiatry Rep 2018;19(12):92.
22. Bejerot S. An autistic dimension: a proposed subtype of obsessive-compulsive disorder. Autism 2007;11(2):101–10.
23. Zaboski BA, Storch EA. Comorbid autism spectrum disorder and anxiety disorders: a brief review. Future Neurol 2018;13(1):31–7.
24. Zandt F, Prior M, Kyrios M. Repetitive behaviour in children with high functioning autism and obsessive compulsive disorder. J Autism Dev Disord 2007;37:251–9.
25. Spiker MA, Lin CE, Marilyn VD, et al. Restricted interests and anxiety in children with autism. Autism 2012;16(3):306–20.
26. Ekman E, Hiltunen AJ. The cognitive profile of persons with obsessive compulsive disorder with and without autism spectrum disorder. Clin Pract Epidemiol Ment Health 2018;14:304–11.

27. Mercier C, Mottron L, Belleville S. A psychosocial study on restricted interests in high-functioning persons with pervasive developmental disorders. Autism 2000; 4(4):406–25.

28. Paula-Perez I. Differential Diagnosis between obsessive compulsive disorder and restrictive and repetitive behavioural patterns, activities, and interests in autism spectrum disorders. Rev Psiquiatr Salud Ment 2013;6(4):178–86.

29. Ruta L, Mugno D, D'Arrigo VG, et al. Obsessive-compulsive traits in children and adolescents with Asperger syndrome. Eur Child Adolesc Psychiatry 2010;19: 17–24.

30. Schaill L, Challa SA. Repetitive behavior in children with autism spectrum disorder: similarities and differences with obsessive-compulsive disorder. In: Mazzone L, Vitiello B, editors. Psychiatric symptoms and comorbidities in autism spectrum disorder. Springer; 2016. p. 39–50.

31. Chok JT, Koesler B. Distinguishing obsessive-compulsive behavior from stereotypy: a preliminary investigation. Behav Modif 2014;38(3):344–73.

32. Bishop SL, Hus V, Duncan A, et al. Subcategories of restricted and repetitive behaviors in children with autism spectrum disorders. J Autism Dev Disord 2013;43: 1287–97.

33. Leyfer O, Folstein S, Bacalman S, et al. Comorbid psychiatric disorders in children with autism: interview development and rates of disorder. J Autism Dev Disord 2006;36:849–61.

34. McDougle CJ, Kresch LE, Goodman WK, et al. A case-controlled study of repetitive thoughts and behaviour in adults with autistic disorder and obsessive-compulsive disorder. Am J Psychiatry 1995;152(5):772–7.

35. Russell AJ, Mataix-Cols D, Anson M, et al. Obsessions and compulsions in Asperger syndrome and high-functioning autism. Br J Psychiatry 2005;186:525–8.

36. Rodgers J, Glod M, Connolly B, et al. The Relationship between anxiety and repetitive behaviours in autism spectrum disorder. J Autism Dev Disord 2012;42: 2404–9.

37. Cath DC, Ran N, Smit JH, et al. Symptom overlap between autism spectrum disorders, generalized social anxiety disorder and obsessive-compulsive disorder in adults: a preliminary case-controlled study. Psychopathology 2008;41:101–10.

38. Lewin AB, Wood JJ, Gunderson S, et al. Phenomenology of comorbid autism spectrum and obsessive-compulsive disorders among children. J Dev Phys Disabil 2011;23:543–53.

39. Buissonniere-Ariza V, Wood JJ, Kendall PC, et al. Presentation and correlates of hoarding behaviors in children with autism spectrum disorders and comorbid anxiety or obsessive-compulsive symptoms. J Autism Dev Disord 2018;48: 4167–78.

40. Cadman T, Spain D, Johnston P, et al, AIMS Consortium. Obsessive-compulsive disorder in adults with high-functioning autism spectrum disorder: what does self-report with the OCI-R tell us? Autism Res 2015;8:477–85.

41. MacNeil BM, Lopes VA, Minnes PM. Anxiety in children and adolescents with autism spectrum disorders. Res Autism Spectr Disord 2009;3:1–21.

42. Humble M, Bejerot S, Bergovist PB, et al. Reactivity of Serotonin in the whole blood: relationship with drug response in obsessive-compulsive disorder. Biol Psychiatry 2001;49(4):360–8.

43. Kose LK, Fox L, Storch EA. Effectiveness of cognitive behavioral therapy for individuals with autism spectrum disorders and comorbid obsessive-compulsive disorder: a review of the research. J Dev Phys Disabil 2018;30(1):69–87.

44. Vause T, Neil N, Jaksie H, et al. Preliminary randomized trial of function-based cognitive-behavioral therapy to treat obsessive compulsive behavior in children with autism spectrum disorder. Focus Autism Other Dev Disabl 2015;32(3):1–11.

45. Wolters LH, de Haan E, Hogendoorn SM, et al. Severe pediatric obsessive compulsive disorder and co-morbid autistic symptoms: effectiveness of cognitive behavioral therapy. J Obsessive Compuls Relat Disord 2016;10:69–77.

46. Iniesta-Sepulveda M, Nadeau JM, Ramos A, et al. An initial case series of intensive cognitive-behavioral therapy for obsessive-compulsive disorder in adolescents with autism spectrum disorder. Child Psychiatry Hum Dev 2018;49:9–19.

47. Russell AJ, Jassi A, Fullana MA, et al. Cognitive behavior therapy for comorbid obsessive-compulsive disorder in high-functioning autism spectrum disorders: a randomized controlled trial. Depress Anxiety 2013;30(8):697–708.

48. Boyd BA, Woodard CR, Bodfish JW. Feasibility of exposure response prevention to treat repetitive behaviors of children with autism and an intellectual disability: a brief report. Autism 2013;17:196–204.

49. Murray K, Jassi A, Mataix-Cols D, et al. Outcomes of cognitive behaviour therapy for obsessive-compulsive disorder in young people with and without autism spectrum disorders: a case controlled study. Psychiatry Res 2015;228:8–13.

50. March JS, Franklin M, Nelson A, et al. Cognitive-behavioral psychotherapy for pediatric obsessive-compulsive disorder. J Clin Child Psychol 2001;30:8–18.

51. Piacentini J, Langley AK. Cognitive-behavioral therapy for children who have obsessive-compulsive disorder. J Clin Psychol 2004;60:1181–94.

52. Lehmkuhl HD, Storch EA, Bodfish JW, et al. Brief Report: exposure and response prevention for obsessive compulsive disorder in a 12-year-old with autism. J Autism Dev Disord 2008;38:977–81.

53. Krebs G, Murray K, Jassi A. Modified cognitive behavior therapy for severe, treatment-resistant obsessive-compulsive disorder in an adolescent with autism spectrum disorder. J Clin Psychol 2016;72(11):1162–73.

54. Marcus RN, Owen R, Kame L, et al. A placebo-controlled, fixed-dose study of aripiprazole in children and adolescents with irritability associated with autistic disorder. J Am Acad Child Adolesc Psychiatry 2009;48(11):1110–9.

55. Owen R, Sikich L, Marcus RN, et al. Aripiprazole in the treatment of irritability in children and adolescents with autistic disorder. Pediatrics 2009;124(6):1533–40.

56. McDougle CJ, Scahill L, Aman MG, et al. Risperidone for the core symptom domains of autism: results from the study by the autism network of the research unit on pediatric psychopharmacology. Am J Psychiatry 2005;162(6):1142–8.

57. Hirsch LE, Pringsheim T. Aripiprazole for autism spectrum disorders (ASD). Cochrane Database Syst Rev 2016;(6):CD00943.

58. Jesner OS, Aref-Adib M, Coren E, et al. Risperidone for autism spectrum disorder. Cochrane Database Syst Rev 2007;(1):CD005040.

59. McDougle CJ, Holmes JP, Carlson DC, et al. A double-blind, placebo-controlled study of risperidone in adults with autistic disorder and other pervasive developmental disorders. Arch Gen Psychiatry 1998;55(7):633–41.

60. Pediatric OCD Treatment Study (POTS) Team. Cognitive-behavior therapy, sertraline, and their combination for children and adolescents with obsessive-compulsive disorder. JAMA 2004;292(16):1969–76.

61. Skapinakis P, Caldwell DM, Hollingworth W, et al. Pharmacological and psychotherapeutic interventions for management of obsessive-compulsive disorder in adults: a systematic review and network meta-analysis. Lancet Psychiatry 2016;3(8):730–9.

62. King BH, Hollander E, Sikich L, et al. Lack of efficacy of citalopram in children with autism spectrum disorders and high levels of repetitive behavior. Arch Gen Psychiatry 2009;66(6):583–90.

63. Hollander E, Phillips A, Chaplin W, et al. A placebo controlled crossover trial of liquid fluoxetine on repetitive behaviors in childhood and adolescent autism. Neuropsychopharmacology 2005;30:582–9.

64. Herscu P, Handen BL, Arnold LE, et al, Murphy and Autism Speaks Autism Clinical Trials Network. The SOFIA Study: negative multi-center study of low dose fluoxetine on repetitive behaviors in children and adolescents with autistic disorder. J Autism Dev Disord 2019. https://doi.org/10.1007/s10803-019-04120-y.

65. McDougle CJ, Kresch LE, Posey DJ. Repetitive thoughts and behavior in pervasive developmental disorders: treatment with serotonin reuptake inhibitors. J Autism Dev Disord 2000;30(5):427–35.

66. McDougle C, Naylor S, Cohen D, et al. A double-blind, placebo controlled study of fluvoxamine in adults with autistic disorder. Arch Gen Psychiatry 1996;53(11): 1001–8.

67. Gordon CT, State RC, Nelson JE, et al. A double-blind comparison of clomipramine, desipramine, and placebo in the treatment of autistic disorder. Arch Gen Psychiatry 1993;50:441–7.

68. Doshi P, Hegde A, Desai A. Nucleus accumbens deep brain stimulation for obsessive-compulsive disorder and aggression in an autistic patient: a case report and hypothesis of the role of the nucleus accumbens in autism and comorbid symptoms. World Neurosurg 2019;125:387–91.

69. Esbensen AJ, Seltzer MM, Lam KS, et al. Age-related differences in restricted repetitive behaviors in autism spectrum disorders. J Autism Dev Disord 2009;39: 57–66.

70. Dold M, Aigner M, Lanzenberger R, et al. Antipsychotic augmentation of serotonin reuptake inhibitors in treatment-resistant obsessive-compulsive disorder: an update meta-analysis of double-blind, randomized placebo-controlled trials. Int J Neuropsychopharmacol 2015;18(9) [pii:pyv047].

71. Arumugham SS, Reddy JY. Augmentation strategies in obsessive-compulsive disorder. Expert Rev Neurother 2013;13(2):187–202.

72. Bolton PF, Pickles A, Murphy M, et al. Autism, affective, and other psychiatric disorders: patterns of familial aggregation. Psychol Med 1998;28:385–95.

73. Carlisi CO, Norman L, Murphy CM, et al, MRC AIMS Consortium. Disorder-specific and shared brain Abnormalities during vigilance in autism and obsessive-compulsive disorder. Biol Psychiatry Cogn Neurosci Neuroimaging 2017;2(8): 644–54.

74. Tsuchiyagaito A, Hirano Y, Asano K, et al. Cognitive-behavioral therapy for obsessive-compulsive disorder with and without autism spectrum disorder: gray matter differences associated with poor outcome. Front Psychiatry 2017; 8:143.

75. Carlisi CO, Norman LJ, Lukito SS, et al. Comparative multimodal meta-analysis of structural and functional brain abnormalities in autism spectrum disorder and obsessive-compulsive disorder. Biol Psychiatry 2017;82:83–102.

76. Akkermans SE, Rheinheimer N, Bruchhage MM, et al, Oldehinkel and TACTICS consortium. Frontostriatal functional connectivity correlates with repetitive behavior across autism spectrum disorder and obsessive-compulsive disorder. Psychol Med 2019;49(13):2247–55.

77. Naaijen J, Zwiers MP, Forde NJ, et al, The TACTICS Consortium. Striatal structure and its association with N-Acetylaspartate and glutamate in autism spectrum

disorder and obsessive compulsive disorder. Eur Neuropsychopharmacol 2018; 28:118–29.

78. Aoki Y, Kasai K, Yamasue H. Age-related change in brain metabolite abnormalities in autism: a meta-analysis of proton magnetic resonance spectroscopy studies. Transl Psychiatry 2012;2(1):e69.

79. Aoki Yuta, Aoki Ai, Suwa H. Reduction of N-acetylaspartate in the medial prefrontal cortex correlated with symptom severity in obsessive-compulsive disorder: meta-analyses of H-MRS studies. Transl Psychiatry 2012;2(8):e153.

80. Naaijen J, Zwiers MP, Amiri H, et al. Fronto-striatal glutamate in autism spectrum disorder and obsessive compulsive disorder. Neuropsychopharmacology 2017; 42:2456–65.

81. Alonso P, Gartacos M, Segalas C, et al. Association between the NMDA glutamate receptor GRIN2B gene and obsessive-compulsive disorder. J Psychiatry Neurosci 2012;37:273–81.

82. Mattila M, Hurtig T, Happsamo H, et al. Comorbid psychiatric disorders associated with Asperger syndrome/high-functioning autism: a community and clinic-based study. J Autism Dev Disord 2010;40:1080–93.

83. Mazefsky CA, Kao J, Oswald DP. Preliminary evidence suggesting caution in the use of psychiatric self-report measures with adolescents with high-functioning autism spectrum disorders. Res Autism Spectr Disord 2011;5(1):164–74.

84. Jacob S, Landeros-Weisenberger A, Leckman JF. Autism spectrum and obsessive-compulsive disorders: OC behaviors, phenotypes and genetics. Autism Res 2009;2:293–311.

85. Ozaki N, Goldman D, Kaye WH, et al. Serotonin transporter missense mutation associated with a complex neuropsychiatric phenotype. Mol Psychiatry 2003;8: 933–6.

86. Bloch MH, Landeros-Weisenberger A, Sen S, et al. Association of the serotonin transporter polymorphism and obsessive-compulsive disorder: systematic review. Am J Med Genet B Neuropsychiatr Genet 2008;147B:850–8.

87. Sagar A, Pinto D, Najjar F, et al. De Novo unbalanced translocation (4p duplication/8p deletion) in a patient with autism, OCD, and overgrowth syndrome. Am J Med Genet A 2017;173(6):1656–62.

88. Alarcon M, Cantor RM, Liu J, et al. Evidence for a language quantitative trait locus on chromosome 7q in multiplex autism families. Am J Hum Genet 2002;70:60–71.

89. Buxbaum JD, Silverman J, Keddache M, et al. Linkage analysis for autism in a subset families with obsessive-compulsive behaviors: evidence for an autism susceptibility gene on chromosome 1 and further support for susceptibility genes on chromosome 6 and 19. Mol Psychiatry 2004;9:144–50.

90. Shao Y, Cuccaro ML, Hauser ER, et al. Fine mapping of autistic disorder to chromosome 15q11-q13 by use of phenotypic subtypes. Am J Hum Genet 2003;72: 539–48.

91. Kuno M, Hirano Y, Nakagawa A, et al. White matter features associated with autistic traits in obsessive-compulsive disorder. Front Psychiatry 2018;9.

92. Hartley SL, Sikora DM. Which DSM-IV-TR criteria best differentiate high-functioning autism spectrum disorder from ADHD and anxiety disorders in older children? Autism 2009;13:485–509.

93. Militerni R, Bravaccio C, Falco C, et al. Repetitive behaviors in autistic disorder. Eur Child Adolesc Psychiatry 2002;11:210–8.

94. South M, Ozonoff S, Mcmahon WM. The relationship between executive functioning, central coherence, and repetitive behaviors in the high-functioning spectrum. Autism 2007;11(5):437–51.

95. Lopez BR, Lincoln AJ, Ozonoff S, et al. Examining the relationship between executive functions and the restricted, repetitive symptoms of autistic disorder. J Autism Dev Disord 2005;35:245–60.
96. Purcell R, Maruff P, Kyrios M, et al. Neuropsychological deficits in obsessive-compulsive disorder: a comparison with unipolar depression, panic disorder, and normal controls. Arch Gen Psychiatry 1998;55(5):415–23.
97. Reaven J, Heburn S. Cognitive-behavioral treatment of obsessive compulsive disorder in a child with Asperger syndrome. Autism 2003;7:145–64.
98. Jassi AD, Kolvenbach S, Heyman I, et al. Increasing knowledge about obsessive compulsive disorder and support for parents and schools: evaluation of initiatives. Health Education 2015;75(5):600–9.

Moving?

Make sure your subscription moves with you!

To notify us of your new address, find your **Clinics Account Number** (located on your mailing label above your name), and contact customer service at:

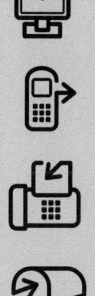

Email: journalscustomerservice-usa@elsevier.com

800-654-2452 (subscribers in the U.S. & Canada)
314-447-8871 (subscribers outside of the U.S. & Canada)

Fax number: 314-447-8029

Elsevier Health Sciences Division
Subscription Customer Service
3251 Riverport Lane
Maryland Heights, MO 63043

*To ensure uninterrupted delivery of your subscription, please notify us at least 4 weeks in advance of move.

Printed and bound by CPI Group (UK) Ltd, Croydon, CR0 4YY

03/10/2024

01040400-0018